The Complete Smith Machine

Exercises & Workouts

Craig Cecil

The Complete Smith Machine: Exercises & Workouts

ISBN: 978-0-9847414-2-7
ISBN: 978-0-9847414-3-4 (ebook)

First edition: July 2013

Manufactured in the United States of America

Trademarked names may appear in this book. Rather than use a trademark symbol with every occurrence of a trademarked name, we use the names only in an editorial fashion and to the benefit of the trademark owner, with no intention of infringement of the trademark.

Warning: This book stresses the importance of proper technique and safety when using bodybuilding and strength training programs. Regardless of your age, before beginning any exercise program consult with your physician to ensure that you are in proper health and that it is appropriate for you to follow such programs. Proceed with caution and at your own risk. This book does not provide medical or therapeutic advice; you should obtain medical advice from your healthcare practitioner. Before starting any new exercise program, check with your doctor, especially if you have a specific physical problem or are taking any medication. The author, publisher or distributors of this book cannot be responsible for any injury, loss or damage caused, or allegedly caused, directly or indirectly, from following the instruction given in this book.

Cover design by Jaclyn Urlahs.

Contents

Thanks!

I want to thank David and Anna for their courage and commitment to pose for the pictures in this book. You can both be proud of your physical achievements and mental fortitude to accomplish that. I know it's not easy putting yourself out there for thousands of readers for eternity. It's also nice to see a husband and wife unified in the pursuit of health, a model which they can pass on to their children. In any case, you have been immortalized.

A special thanks to Mark and Janet for the gracious use of their gym used to shoot all the photos in this book and to Leslie for taking the pictures.

Finally, I want to extend a big thank you to Leslie and Kayleigh for the meticulous grammar-checking, proof-reading, and editing of this book. It really is a lot better book because of your efforts.

Craig

Tell Me What You Think

I'm always interested in getting feedback on my books. Please send your comments and suggestions to:

books@runningdeersoftware.com

Each man delights in the work that suits him best.

— Homer, *The Odyssey*

Preface

The Smith Machine is one of the most common and versatile pieces of weight training equipment ever devised, equally effective for both beginners and advanced trainers alike. It was the first true multi-purpose exercise machine and, due to its versatility, is found in gyms, health clubs, schools and homes around the world. Its basic design of a barbell affixed to a sliding rail system allows for the safe use of pushing and pulling exercises with light to heavy weights. However, perhaps due to its deceptively simple design, the Smith Machine is often relegated to simple squats, shrugs, and presses. You can work any muscle group on modern versions of the Smith Machine. The collection of basic barbell movements you can do here represents a symphony of exercises that can transform your body.

Additionally, the Smith Machine presents a unique opportunity to enhance your strength, build more muscle, reshape your body, reduce body fat, recover from injuries, and save time working out.

My goal here is two-fold.

First, I hope to show you just about every possible use for the Smith Machine in your training. In that vein, this book presents a complete guide to the *effective* use of the Smith Machine, presenting over 80 exercises and dozens of varied workouts, for the beginner to the advanced trainer. Additionally, the book will show you how to take advantage of the machine's unique strengths, *while avoiding its weaknesses*, to take your body to the next level in strength and fitness. No matter what your level of workout experience, when you finish reading this book, I guarantee you'll have learned something new and perhaps look at the Smith Machine in a different light. There's more than meets the eye here.

Second, I hope to make this book an enjoyable journey for you. For many, the words learning and joy don't often coexist. However, usually the best type of learning is that which we enjoy. I've read hundreds of cookie-cutter fitness books—everything from getting a big bench to fascial stretching, from building massive arms quickly to working out 20 minutes a day, twice per week. At the time, they may have been interesting, but over time most of the contents have slipped the surly bonds of practical use. The ones I hold dearest are peppered with histories, stories, anecdotes and absolute truths I could relate to, perhaps eliciting a grin or laugh, and ultimately etching into long-term memory. I'll try to follow that form—ultimately, you'll decide if I succeeded.

Now, let's start at the beginning.

1

The Soul of a New Machine

I've often been quoted as saying that history holds the key to discovery or re-discovery of physical improvement—those barbells, dumbbells and various tools used in our weight training pursuits have stories to tell that help us understand not only their purpose, but effective use as well. This history holds no less importance to us here with weight training techniques, methodologies and equipment, than does the story of Agamemnon launching the Trojan War to scholars.

No matter which type of fitness routine you follow, whether you use aerobics, recreational weight training, or are involved with serious bodybuilding or powerlifting, the roads to these endeavors typically converge back to Jack LaLanne. Most who remember him will remember the tight, one-piece zippered jump suits he wore when working out on television. Whereas the jumpsuits helped build the brand, he fathered just about everything we now associate with the modern fitness revolution.

Starting in the 1950s, LaLanne pioneered physical fitness and nutrition through an array of venues—early television (aspiring cooks had Julia Child—exercise buffs had *The Jack LaLanne Show*), books, one of the first health club chains, personal training of celebrities—along with incredible feats of strength, such as swimming a mile in Long Beach Harbor, while handcuffed and shackled, towing 13 boats containing 76 people—at 62 years old. He also invented a number of exercise machines—which brings us here.

In the early 1950s, Lalanne wanted an exercise machine that would provide the benefits of free-weight workouts to a wider audience, with as much built-in safety as possible. That was always his goal—to get people up off the couch and exercising and he did anything he could to further that aim. Jack rigged up a simple prototype of his "free weight" machine in his gym. The prototype had sliding rails, extending from floor to ceiling that acted as guides for the attached barbell. Now, even novice weight trainers could safely perform simple pressing and pulling exercises, without worrying about balancing or falling over with the bar (it happens). It seemed like a great way to get even more people working out.

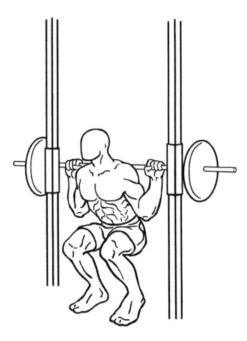

Artist rendering of Jack LaLanne's early rail-based exercise machine

Rudy Smith thought it was a great idea too. It just needed a few modifications.

Rudy was a bodybuilder working out at LaLanne's gym in the early 1950s when Jack constructed his prototype. Realizing its potential, Rudy continued modifying the original design on his own so that it could be free standing—the rails would not be affixed to floor and ceiling—and could accommodate heavier loads, provide smoother operation through a counter-weight system, and have safety catches negating the need for a spotter. Rudy Smith's final design incorporated all of these modifications, using dumbbell plates attached to bicycle chains as the counter-weight mechanism.

By then, Rudy was working as the manager of the Vic Tanny gym in Los Angeles and had his Smith Machine installed for the members to use. The machine was an instant hit, more machines were ordered and installed in all the Vic Tanny gyms, word quickly spread, and several other health club chains inquired about getting their own.

Due to the overwhelming demand, Smith hired the machinist Paul Martin to design a version that could be mass-produced. At the time, Martin was pioneering the genesis of the commercial health club equipment industry, supplying the Vic Tanny and Ray Wilson's American Health Studio chains with early fitness equipment from his factory. This Rudy Smith/Paul Martin collaboration produced the original edition of the mass market Smith Machine—the basic design still in use today.

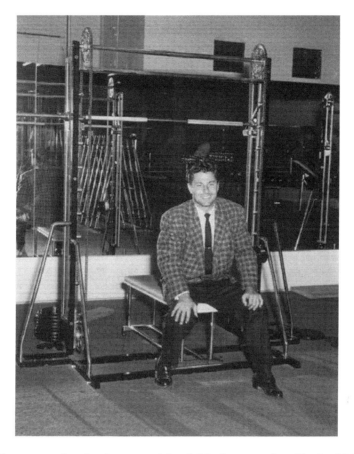

Vic Tanny seated under the original Smith Machine, produced by Paul Martin

2

Meet the Smith Machine

The modern Smith Machine, found in most health clubs and available for home gym use, is virtually unchanged from Rudy Smith's original manufactured unit. The proven design produces results.

Today, Smith Machines are available in two general versions—traditional and angled.

The traditional version is the simplest and still uses the purely vertical bar path of the original, and may or may not have a counter-weight mechanism. This version is best for strict vertical motions, such as deadlifts, rows and squats.

Angled versions are either counter-weighted or use a viscous resistance for smooth operation, and are typically set at a 7-10 degree incline, allowing a more natural movement for presses, upright rows and shrugs, expanding the available sandbox of movements over the traditional version.

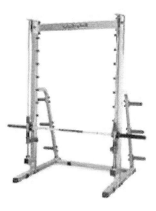 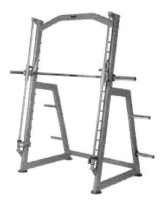

Although fairly uncommon, some newer design Smith Machines do allow a limited horizontal movement, as well as the vertical bar path. Because these machines are so uncommon, you're not likely to find one at your local gym. However, if you do have access to one of these, all of the information in this book still applies—you'll just have a little more freedom of motion, which is never a bad thing.

Regardless of the type of Smith Machine you have access to, the basic operation and safety features remain the same. The affixed barbell contains a built-in hook mechanism on each side of the bar. You lift the bar and twist it backward to unhook (unlock) it from the post or slot that currently holds it in place (some machines reverse this operation and have you twist the bar forward to unlock). This allows the bar to move freely along the rails. When you want to secure the barbell, you can twist the bar forward at any point in order to hook it into the nearest post or slot.

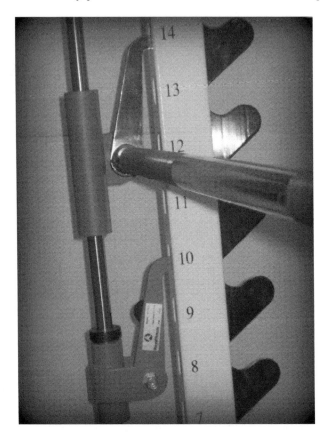

The hook locking mechanism (top) and the safety catch (bottom)

Additionally, before you begin the exercise you can adjust the moveable safety guards that slide along each rail. These safety guards will stop the descent of the bar in the event that you are unable to twist the barbell into place with heavy loads. These guards are also the key to setting the desired range of motion for your chosen exercise.

The only two things you have to remember when using the Smith Machine are to (1) set the safety catches at an appropriate spot in the event you can't complete the movement, and (2) keep the bar rotated in the unlocked position throughout your exercise. It's common for Smith Machine novices to forget to set the safety mechanisms and to inadvertently rotate the bar into the locked position while the bar travels along the rails, making for a jarring experience. However, with a couple minutes of practice, you'll be expert at the operation of the machine. That's the beauty of the design.

That's it folks—a simple machine with a simple operation that allows you to do a vast array of exercises safely. But that's not the end of the story, at least as far as some are concerned...

3

Advantages, Disadvantages & Limitations

The Smith Machine is a controversial device. Depending on who you listen to, it's either the greatest thing since man caught a stick on fire or represents the evil Mephistopheles of weight training. When you ask a seasoned weightlifter what the Smith Machine is useful for, typical answers are "I don't know", "Presses, squats and shrugs", or "as a coat hanger". Like most things, the truth is somewhere in between.

Novices, or those with injuries, are drawn to the machine for its unassuming, easy to operate nature within a safe environment. Exercise scientists, powerlifters, weightlifters, and functional movement experts denounce the machine for its limitations and potential for harm—opting instead to urge all of us to focus our efforts on free-weight and body-based movements. For the sheer act of writing this book, these groups may initially brand me as ignorant, traitorous or a snake oil salesman. Who is right? Let's find out.

Advantages

On the surface, the obvious advantages the Smith Machine offers are:

Self-spotting

Because the machine offers both safety catches and the ability to lock the bar in place by simply rotating it, there is no need for a spotter when performing exercises with heavy weights, such as squats and presses. This can allow advanced trainers to push themselves without fear. It's also vitally important if you want to achieve muscle growth—muscles must be forced into growth by making them perform things (more weight, more reps) they haven't done before. The Smith Machine gives you the confidence to do this. And let's face it—most people work out by themselves, whether at home or the gym. It's next to impossible to find a good, consistent training partner, so when you want to push yourself, self-spotting starts to look real good.

Balance & Stability

You don't need to balance the bar when using the Smith Machine; therefore you can't fall forward, back or sideways—again providing confidence. This allows novice trainers to concentrate more on form, without the worry of balance and stability. It also provides you an environment where as little can go wrong as possible. Besides getting in shape, workout novices also don't want to look stupid. If you've never used free weights before, they can make you look stupid, due to your lack of balance and stability when learning a new movement. If the Smith Machine gets you past the initial fear of stupidity, more power to it.

For trainers with a little more experience, if you can't "feel" the muscle working with a free weight movement, try performing the exercise on the Smith Machine, if possible. Just the pure concentration on form may allow you to make that mind/muscle connection that's so important for progress. In this situation, the Smith Machine's balance and stability becomes a pattern-based learning tool.

Whereas self-spotting and built-in balance and stability are obvious benefits, there are some less obvious ones as well:

Provides a Transition to Free Weights

Let's just state this now—free weights rule in the world of weight training. That's eventually where you want to be. However, the vast majority of people who start going to the gym or start training at home to get off the couch and get in better shape, don't start with free weights. Why?—because they don't know how and are afraid.

Many people are just plain intimidated by free weights or those of who have used free weights for a while. In a Darwinian world, this is natural. As mentioned above, the Smith Machine can help you climb that evolutionary ladder, by providing confidence and a natural bridge from using machines to the promised land of free weights.

Initially, the machine gets you familiar with loading plates on a bar. That's a big first step, especially for those accustomed to setting their weight resistance by placing a pin in a machine's weight stack. This gentle familiarity is also one reason why plate-loaded equipment, such as Hammer Strength, is so popular in gym and fitness centers today.

Second, you get used to gripping and holding onto an Olympic bar—you know, the ones they use in the actual Olympics for weightlifting and use as standardized equipment in all gyms across the world, regardless of race, religion, nationality or measurement unit. The Olympic bar is the Rosetta Stone of resistance training.

Third, the Smith Machine breeds familiarity with free-weight type movements, such as squats, deadlifts and presses when holding onto that Olympic bar. You're halfway home.

Finally, it requires you to make decisions and discover the consequences—such as what weight to use, or how much weight to add to the bar for the next set, the next workout, etc. You have to choose from the 45, 25, 10, 5 and 2.5lb plates—a virtual cornucopia of options that allow for more minute increments in weight versus the unyielding increments of typical machines. You get good at gym math. It's not just about setting the pin in slot number seven on the leg extension machine anymore.

All these things combined—loading plates, using an Olympic bar, patterning new movements and making the same decisions you need to make with free weights provide a great learning transition from pure machine-based workouts to the big time. And your confidence and physique will improve as a result.

Once you eventually make the move to a predominantly free-weight based workout regimen, the Smith Machine still provides a useful alternative in specific situations, as I'll relate later.

Confidence

I mentioned this earlier, but it bears repeating because it's so often overlooked in the pantheon of weight training milieu—anything which provides relative safety, requires minimal balance and stability and has you performing free-weight like movements and activities builds confidence. The converse is also true—it minimizes embarrassment, which let's face it, is one of the big reasons beginners at gyms avoid the free weight area. For exercise-machine devotees, the Smith Machine seems somewhat similar, yet slightly strange—offering an invitation to try it.

The Smith Machine enforces structure. People like structure. And structure builds confidence.

Constant Tension

This isn't often mentioned, but because the Smith Machine provides a linear bar path, it affords the opportunity to enlist constant tension on the muscles being worked when performing an exercise.

For example, because you don't need to concentrate on balance or stability, you can really work on squeezing your pectorals (chest) right from the start when performing incline presses, instead of just myopically pushing your hands toward the ceiling. This technique of keeping the muscle under constant tension (time under load) is one of the great benefits of the machine.

Muscle Isolation

Functional movement experts and many personal trainers talk about working the body as a single unit/system, performing whole body movements or actions that enlist as many muscle groups as possible. There's nothing wrong with that approach—in fact, it's great most of the time.

However, there are times when you need to isolate muscles, perhaps due to asymmetrical development (one arm bigger or stronger than the other), issues with muscle imbalance (large quads, small hamstrings), or injuries. The Smith Machine serves a dual purpose—it provides opportunity to work large groups of muscles at once, or isolate muscles when needed.

For example, on traditional squats, there are typically two types of lifters—what I like to call glute-dominant lifters (they mainly use their butt) and quad-dominant lifters (they primarily use their quadriceps/thighs). A lot of this has to do with technique, and some with body type. The Smith Machine allows these types of issues to be isolated and re-balanced. Glute-dominant lifters can perform squats with their feet slightly forward of the bar, shifting much of the work from the glutes to the thighs, without fear of falling. Further, lifters with minor back issues can often position their backs in a more vertical orientation in the Smith Machine and still squat, despite the injury. Many lifters who can't perform free weight squats, due to past back injuries, often thrive with Smith Machine squats. That's just one example. There are countless more.

(Limited) Range of Motion

The ability to exact control (set limits) on the range of motion is beneficial in certain circumstances. Because you can set the safety mechanism on the Smith Machine to restrict your range of motion, you have a confident means of working an area through a restricted range. This allows strength athletes to work with supramaximal loads.

Some individuals can't use free weights without incurring pain—minor stability or bar path changes can aggravate shoulder, back, neck or joints. Older lifters often have joint (arthritis, tendonitis) or mobility issues. Slight to moderate constraints on the range of motion with specific exercises can allow these individuals to continue training and improving their bodies.

Disadvantages & Limitations

Most of the arguments surrounding the disadvantages of the Smith Machine are rooted in its physical design limitations. Let's take a look at those.

Fixed Plane of Motion

Because the Smith Machine's bar can only move up and down, limiting the body to a fixed plane of motion, experts argue that it's unnatural and dangerous for the body to move this way, given that many exercises exhibit a natural arc of movement. The emanation from this camp is that the Smith Machine can increase the risk of injury, especially to the knees and lower back.

However, a consensus of scientific evidence in support of this is lacking, whereas the practicum of bodybuilders over the decades have discovered that fixed planes can be excellent for hammering a muscle into submission. On the other hand, the Olympic lifts (snatch, clean and jerk) do require arc-based movements and cannot be performed on the Smith Machine. Another valid consideration is that traditional weight lifting movements that can include a slight natural arc, such as the bench press and squat, will experience a loss of force as the Smith Machine bar travels through that fixed plane. It's just simple physics. I'll tell you why that's important in a minute.

Lack of Stabilizer Muscle Activation

This argument goes hand in hand with a fixed plane of motion. Any time you have a fixed plane many of your stabilizer muscles are not actively recruited. Why is this important? Read on.

Does not Improve Coordination & Balance

OK. Because the Smith Machine has a fixed plane, which doesn't actively use your stabilizer muscles, what's the repercussion? It doesn't improve your coordination and balance—two keys to overall fitness. For athletes, improving coordination and balance are part of the total package for improving performance. Again, context is paramount—for bodybuilders, the Smith Machine provides many benefits; for a baseball or football player, not so much.

However, as I've mentioned, there are times you may not want to involve your stabilizer muscles. For example, many individuals have trouble building the upper chest because their front deltoids (shoulders) take the brunt of the work (next time you perform ten sets of bench presses, a day or two later notice how sore your chest is compared to your front delts—if only your front delts are sore, pay attention to the next sentence). Some of this is due to structural genetics (wide clavicles, shallow ribcage) or exercise set-up and performance (incline set too high, shoulders do not remain retracted). If this is you, performing incline presses on the Smith Machine will allow you to set your body and the movement in a position to help you primarily work your upper chest and not your shoulders.

Transfer of Skills

Physical tasks are not performed in a linear fixed plane. Your body doesn't move that way. As many exercise scientists point out, because Smith Machine exercises do not mimic most physical tasks they are less functional than free weight versions. This is just the bare truth. Be aware of it, because your body will be. The take away message is that there is no silver bullet, whether it is barbells, dumbbells, cables, sandbags, Husafell Stones, or Smith Machines.

◆ ◆ ◆ ◆

The basic problem with arguments centering on the Smith Machine's disadvantages is they are often arguments in a vacuum, mutually exclusive, all-or-nothing arguments. If you are going to use the Smith Machine exclusively as your only weight-training device, then yes, you will be limited to a fixed plane, which requires you to exempt some movements—and compared to others who perform mostly free weight movements, you will be at a disadvantage.

However, that's not the raison d'être of the machine. Jack LaLanne's original intent for the machine still applies—to get more people exercising. If the Smith Machine gets you up off the couch, gets you back in the game from an injury, saves you a little time, and opens your world to more exercises, then so be it. Look around at the mass of humanity—it's better than the alternative.

What we really need is to derive maximum benefit from the machine.

Given the inherent advantages, disadvantages and limitations described above, you need to understand how to use the Smith Machine *effectively* in order to derive maximum benefit. The Smith Machine is simply one tool in your overall fitness arsenal to achieve your physical goals. The next section shows you how to use this tool based on your specific goals, to produce maximum benefit.

4

How to Use the Smith Machine Effectively

All weight training activities lie on a continuum, from explosive, violent single-rep power movements to the grace and fluidity of high-volume, minimal rest circuit training. Each waypoint along that progression has distinct effects on the body. This section will introduce you to those waypoints. Regardless of where you are or where you want to proceed along this weight training continuum, lifting weights is an exceptional activity to gain muscle, lose fat and increase joint mobility.

For most, the Smith Machine equates to various presses, squats, and perhaps shrugs. Typical use is generally a couple sets of each of those movements for 6-12 reps, with about a minute or two of rest in between. Folks, that's just the tip of the iceberg here. Basic barbell movements represent a symphony of exercises that transform your body—affixing a barbell to a rail system hardly detracts from that.

When people work out, they usually have at least a loosely defined goal of where they want to be, what they want to achieve—get stronger, build some muscle, lose some fat, or fix some problem areas. Some just need to focus on one or two of those goals—others all of them. But for most, the task set before them is similar to that faced by Odysseus—they just don't know how to get there.

Each of those goals requires following a different path—a significantly different application of progressive-resistance weight training. However, no matter the method you choose, several universal principles apply to any weight training endeavor—get stronger, identify and prioritize weaknesses, learn to deal with and recover from injuries, and the consistency of effort. Above all else, consistency is king. Have the courage to pick one type of training, stick to it for a reasonable length of time, and see where it leads. Call it persistence, stubbornness, or unyielding determination, the unwavering hand is often the hand of the victor. (Somehow, the steel and iron used in weight training never fails to reveal the inherent amount of steel and iron of character within you.) The remainder of this book will describe how you can incorporate the Smith Machine into application of these principles along the continuum within a sensible weight-training program that fits your goals. By the end, you should be able to get from where you are now to the actualization of where you want to be.

Right off the bat, I want to impart two messages. First, this book is aimed at two audiences. The relative beginners to weight-training who may have access to a Smith Machine as their only means of weight training (think home users) or have only used selectorized weight-stack type machines at a gym; and experienced weight trainers who are looking for something that can aid in their quest. I don't want you to think that I offer a silver bullet in the form of a Smith Machine as your physique salvation. I'm just trying to build your toolbox here and widen that universe.

Second, and this goes out to all the women reading this—don't skip past the strength training and bodybuilding sections. As nature has dictated, by performing those types of training you won't inadvertently transform yourself into some manly creature, any more than you can transform a fat molecule into a strand of muscle fiber. The female body just doesn't have the natural testosterone to build the body of a man or anything close to that. The image you may hold of typical female powerlifters or bodybuilders is due to their use of male hormones (steroids), lousy diet, and an unforgivingly myopic focus. On the contrary, women who incorporate strength training and bodybuilding into their overall fitness routines accentuate what makes a woman a woman. Suddenly, you have shapely thighs, nice calves and a great butt, not to mention a tight waist and arms, strong shoulders and back. Think Sigourney Weaver in *Aliens*, Linda Hamilton in *Terminator 2*, or Scarlett Johansson in *The Avengers* for a more accurate picture.

Finally, don't forget that all of the methods, techniques and exercises presented in the remainder of this book apply equally to barbell and dumbbell training.

In that vein, let's briefly visit each stop on this weight training continuum—at each juncture, the Smith Machine has a use, purpose and effect. (I'll get into much more detail about how to perform each type of training in the workout section). Success at any point depends on your integrity, consistency, honesty, intelligence and desire.

Strength Training

If you don't know where to start, start with strength. Getting stronger will help you with any of your physique goals. Think of it this way—if you are building a house that you want to live in for a long time, you need to start with a solid foundation. If you like living in big houses, strength training will allow you to lay that large foundation. If you don't like that well-worn analogy, then think of it this way—it'll make every physical activity you do in your life easier. Strength training's main purpose is to get you stronger than you are now, both physically *and mentally*. (We often forget the mental benefits.) What you do with that strength is up to you. Besides improving muscular strength, this type of training increases bone density, strengthens your tendons and ligaments and conditions your central nervous system to move heavy things. Get good at strength training and you can erect all kinds of stuff on that foundation (bodybuilding, circuit training, athletics, etc.) with no problem.

Traditional strength training workouts are characterized by a few compound, multi-joint movements (squats, deadlifts, cleans, rows, presses), using heavy weights, relatively few sets and ample rest times (2-5 minutes) between those sets for recovery. The workouts are often brief, intense and taxing. Common workout schemes include performing five sets of five reps for each exercise, and working out three times per week in a heavy, medium and light fashion. In the strength training workouts presented later, I'll provide more specifics about the nuances of these options.

Because the weights used are so heavy, most traditional strength training is performed with a barbell and a power rack for safety. For those without that barbell/power rack combo who want to increase their strength, the Smith Machine does offer a good alternative, allowing you to use supra-heavy loads and work within specific ranges of motion. When you are handling weights that you can only lift for 1-5 reps, adherence to proper form is essential.

These are the bare-bones basics of strength training. They're time-tested over the past century, they won't fail you (if you don't fail them) and they just plain work. However, if you have a thirst for more in-depth knowledge in this area (and I hope you do), I encourage you to check out the writings of Dan John, Mark Rippetoe, and Bill Starr, to name a few.

Bodybuilding

If strength training can produce the Farnese Hercules, then bodybuilding gives birth to Michelangelo's David. As Charles Atlas showed us almost a hundred years ago, this is where most guys dream to be—adding significant muscle mass to their body, whether chest, shoulders, arms or legs. Hopefully, along with muscle size, they are considering symmetry and proportion as well, although from decades of experience in weight rooms, Mr. Upper Body America seems to dominate significantly. We're talking hypertrophy-based bodybuilding here folks. This is also where mirrors rule and pants don't lie. Now would be a good time to stop drinking a gallon of whole milk a day, but that's a story for another time. This is also the type of training along the weight lifting continuum that some people refer to when speaking of "toning up", "body sculpting", or "shaping up". They may not realize it, but that's bodybuilding training.

Although strength training's main purpose is to get you stronger, it will also help you get more muscular. Think of strength training as bodybuilding's older brother with a different attitude (you both do share much of the same DNA)—the older brother may not necessarily care what he looks like, just that he can keep pounding his little brother into the ground whenever he wants. However, while little brother may eventually get all the attention due to his general appearance, he really does need his big strength training brother to help him get there.

That may be an oversimplified and stereotypical analogy, but it's essentially what we are talking about here. To build more muscle, re-shape your body or tone up you need to get stronger, but for bodybuilders you have to balance that purpose with the additional goals of symmetry and proportion so the physique has a pleasing aesthetic flow. Here's the assessment rule—if you've put on some significant muscle mass and then ask someone to identify your most prominent muscle group(s) and they can't decide, you know you've succeeded—that's symmetry. The symmetrical, proportioned physique has no dominant muscle groups and no glaring weaknesses (if only we could all be so lucky, which is the reason for the next section on Weak Point Training). Some of you may remember Steve Reeves as Hercules—that's pure symmetry personified.

As we journey along the continuum from pure strength training, bodybuilding-style hypertrophy-based workouts are characterized by an expanded sandbox of movements, a mix of compound and isolation exercises, using moderate weights, low to moderate reps (6-12), with moderate rest intervals (1-3 minutes), and either brief, high-intensity sessions or traditional lower-intensity, longer duration volume-based sessions. You'll notice that's a lot of moderation there—whereas strength and circuit-based weight training occupy polar extremes of the weight training strata, bodybuilding workouts tend to fall in the middle. Not too light or too heavy, not a lot of rest but definitely not too little, everything just right, as Goldilocks might say.

Circuit Training

Whereas strength training and bodybuilding improve muscular power and size, circuit training focuses on improving muscular endurance while effecting a higher cardiovascular reaction. Studies at The Cooper Institute have continually shown that circuit training is the most time-effective method for enhancing muscular and cardiovascular endurance at the same time. Like the twelve labors of Hercules, it will test your strength and stamina.

What this means is that with circuit training you'll do a series of exercises (a circuit) using moderate weights and moderate to high repetitions with little to no rest between those exercises. After the circuit is complete, take a brief rest, then either perform that circuit again or start a different circuit. You'll get some weight-bearing exercise while your heart rate rises and remains elevated for the entire workout. This is how the workouts at the Curves™ chain of women's fitness centers operate.

But don't be fooled—just because Curves™ uses this type of training doesn't mean it's just for women, it's less intense or doesn't produce good results. CrossFit™ training takes the circuit training methodology to an entirely new level with circuits composed of Olympic and powerlifting movements, tire flips, and Prowler pushes. It isn't easy. This type of training is also excellent preparation and maintenance conditioning for those in the military, law enforcement and for athletes in general.

With strategic ordering of Smith Machine-based exercises, you can perform circuit training effectively without leaving the confines of the machine and with minimal weight changes between exercises. The circuit training workout section presented later will provide you with a plethora of Smith Machine-based circuits you can try.

Cardiovascular Training

I know what you're thinking. You can't perform cardio work on the Smith Machine—that requires running, jogging, biking, rowing, etc. Yes, you can do those activities. But if you only have about ten minutes to get in an effective cardio session, you might be a little limited there.

Not too long ago, a researcher at the College of Sport and Health Science at Ritsumeikan University discovered that by performing high-intensity intermittent training (HIIT) using anaerobic (weightlifting) exercises you could produce significant cardiovascular effects, including incredible fat burning results. Professor Izumi Tabata was quantifying what many elite athletes, especially those from the former Soviet Eastern Bloc countries, had been practicing for decades—performing short, intense interval training with weights can vastly improve athletic conditioning and make you much leaner.

The Tabata Method encapsulates twenty seconds of ultra-intense exercise, followed by ten seconds of rest, repeated continually within a four minute timeframe. This works best with exercises that involve as many muscles as possible in a single movement, such as deadlifts, squats, cleans, snatches and presses.

Although you can't perform cleans, snatches and some other arcing movements on the Smith Machine, you can use it to effectively perform Tabata squats, front squats, deadlifts, RDLs, military presses, etc. The cardio workout section presented later will give you some ideas on this. I guarantee you'll get the same effect here that you do with a long steady-state cardio session.

Weak Point Training

By now, you should notice a process—get stronger, which builds more muscle, which surfaces strengths and weaknesses, which you need to rebalance and correct. That lands you here. Over time, as you get stronger and add some muscle to your body, you'll begin to notice some areas that just don't respond as well as others. This is normal. What happens next is determined by how honest you are with yourself.

Weak point training is the process of balancing your physique, correcting those weak problem areas, and creating a finished proportional, symmetrical masterpiece of you. Except the honest traveler will find the task is never quite finished.

What we need here are specific exercises, techniques and methodologies based on goals, weaknesses and problem areas. For men, this might be more leg size, a wider back or more upper chest. Ladies often complain of unshapely thighs and that thing hanging down from the back of their arms. The section on weak point training workouts presented later will identify these common weaknesses and provide you with a path to correct them using the Smith Machine.

Injury Rehab

Reward and accomplishment require risk. Weight training, in any permutation, is an inherently risky endeavor (as are soccer, basketball, skiing, biking, etc.) and it's virtually impossible to avoid being injured at some point. Whether in the gym or outside of it, eventually a physical or mental lapse will cause something to go awry. Most people don't know how to deal with this, especially the strategy of using specialized weight training to rebuild the injured area.

Because the Smith Machine offers similar benefits to a power rack, especially concerning limiting the range of motion, this can be used to assist in the recovery of many injuries. Coupled with a systematic method of weight, rep and tempo changes, you can heal most acute low back, shoulder, knee and elbow injuries using the Smith Machine as part of your overall rehab strategy.

The Injury Rehab section presented later will detail specifics on how to plan and execute your recovery from these ailments as well as train around them. You may need to swallow your pride during this process (and perhaps hubris got you here in the first place), but the alternative could be much worse—neglecting these injuries often leads to chronic problems which can curtail your weight training career permanently.

Periodization

Regardless of which training path you follow, eventually progress will halt. It's at these times I remember one of the central messages from strength coach Dan John, "Everything works…for about six weeks." In my head, this is followed by the distant voice of former Mr. Olympia Larry Scott saying, "you've gone stale, it's time for change" (and betraying my age, accompanied by the Motley Crüe song of similar name forever etched into my brain during my earliest lifting sessions).

The answer to this is of course, periodization.

This is where the kids would text, "WTF?"

Here are the basics.

Although periodization training has been around since the ancient Greeks prepared for the original Olympic Games, Soviet sport scientist Dmitri Matveyev first formalized the general training concept of periodization (cycle training) in the 1960s, as a method for mapping out the entire year's training program through periods of maximal and submaximal work (intensity). This method is based on the results of scientific research on how best to develop an athlete to his/her fullest potential. The rationale behind periodization is that *you cannot train the same way all the time*. (Read that last sentence again.) To do so will cause stagnation and plateaus in strength, muscle growth, fat loss—basically, everything. I don't know your goals, but I don't think you want this.

By performing different types of weight training over a prolonged period of time you can make steady progress, achieving peak performance, fat loss, conditioning and strength and muscular development at specified times. This helps alleviate boredom and keeps the body adapting. Just keeping yourself interested and motivated to train over a long period of time is the often the biggest hurdle and one of the most important characteristics for success in any fitness-oriented endeavor.

Now, here comes the rub—periodization requires planning. Which is why periodization doesn't work for most—by nature, people aren't planners. But they do like structure.

I'm going to keep this whole thing simple for you. To implement periodization into your fitness schedule, every 6-8 weeks I want you to take a week of active rest (go for a walk, play a little tennis or whatever you might like to do—this is a great time to paint the fence, clean the garage or take mini-vacations with the kids). Then, when you return to the weights, switch to any other type of training listed above (strength training, bodybuilding, weak point training, circuit training) other than the one you just completed—for a few weeks. Repeat this process forever. Now, the catch is you need to intelligently switch from one type of training to another. What does that mean? It means that if your primary goal is to get stronger, then most of the time you need to be strength training. That translates into alternating between strength training for 6-8 weeks, and then some other type of training for a couple weeks, then right back to strength training. The key is that strength training is what you do most of the time. What you don't want to do is just rotate between all different kinds of training. If you do that, you either don't have a plan or don't know what you want. Most people know what they want (they just don't know how to get there or lack the fortitude for the journey). Start there.

This works for anyone, regardless of primary goal. If you fancy yourself a powerlifter and you practice strength training, take that week of active rest, then come back and do some relatively heavy circuit training. For aspiring bodybuilders, you know you need to spend 6-8 weeks fixing your weaknesses with weak point training. In addition, cardio nuts who can't do anything slowly might want to spend the next 6-8 weeks building a stronger foundation with strength training. Believe me, your level of cardio fitness will still be there when you get back—in fact, it should be a lot higher.

◆ ◆ ◆ ◆

The real lesson with periodization and with weight training in general is that not every workout needs to be Armageddon or Sisyphean in nature. Both Icarus and Goldilocks have been telling us this since we were in grade school. Just like your life, there are periods of high stress and relative relaxation. Except here, you get to exert some control when each happens. To wrap up this section, if you ask which type of training is best for you, the answer, in every case, is all of them.

5

The Muscles: What You Need to Know

Let's make sure you understand what the purposes of each of your muscles are before we go any further. I'm still amazed all these years later at how many people in the gym labor away for years without this basic knowledge. Trying to work out without this knowledge is like trying to drive a car when you are eight years old—it can be done, but usually doesn't end well or to your expectations. If you don't have this basic understanding you will never optimize the muscular physique that lies within. It allows you to unlock the code to muscular development.

You may see terms such as flexion, abduction, external rotation, etc. describing how muscles and joints function. In general, I'm not going to use those terms, because you won't remember them, and you probably don't care.

First, let's make sure you know what each muscle is called and where it's located on your body, because you'll need to know this to understand each of the exercises presented later. Then, we'll make sure you know what each muscle (or muscle group) does.

Muscle	Location & Function
Abdominals	Your stomach area—also includes the sides of your stomach (the "love" handles). They are also called "abs".
	Moves your chest towards your waist, flexes the spinal column and lifts the ribs and moves them together.
Back	Everything behind your upper body—also called the "lats" (upper back) and spinal erectors (lower back). Pulls the shoulders down and backwards.

Muscle	Location & Function
Biceps	The front of your upper arm. Lifts and curls the arm and turns the wrist up.
Calves	The back of your lower leg. Flexes the foot.
Chest	You know where this is—also called the pectorals (pecs). Pulls the arms and shoulders across the front of the body.
Forearms	Your lower arm between the elbow and hand. Curls the palm up and down.
Glutes	This is your butt, derrière, tush, or whatever you like to call it. Helps you stand from a seated position, straighten your legs, assist in forward movement, and support your pelvis, lower back and vertebrae. It's the epicenter—the power core of your body and the foundation of your strength.
Hamstrings	The back of your upper leg. Curls the leg back (brings your foot to your butt).
Quadriceps	Your thighs or front of your upper legs—also called "quads". Extends and straightens the leg.
Shoulders	These are the deltoids and are basically made up of front, side and rear parts. Rotates and lifts the arm to the front, side, and rear.
Trapezius	The area beside and behind your neck where you would massage someone—called the "traps". Looks like a small kite attached to your upper back. Raises the shoulders up.
Triceps	The back of your upper arm. Straightens the arm and turns the wrist down.

6

The Exercises

Everything in this section is about moving the bar on the Smith Machine up and down as efficiently as possible, while working as many or as few muscles as indicated.

Ever since the earliest incarnations of man emerging from the primordial swamp, the human body was designed to perform pushing, pulling, squatting and hinge movements, which we can group into the following categories:

Basic Human Movements	
▪ Vertical Pushing	▪ Vertical Pulling
▪ Horizontal Pushing	▪ Vertical Pushing
▪ Squatting	▪ Hip Hinge

In this part of the book, I'll present over 80 exercises which mimic these basic pushing, pulling and hinge movements using the Smith Machine. Sure, you can perform any of these movements with barbells, dumbbells, kettlebells, buckets, rocks, or cans of corn. I hope you try them with any apparatus or implement you have. Basic human movements are basic human movements—the body really doesn't care what you are using. Here, we have a Smith Machine, so we'll use that. Most of the exercises will require you to load plates on the machine and use it directly—others will have you hanging and anchoring yourself using the machine, using it indirectly without the need for plates. If you don't understand any of that, don't worry—I'll explain everything below. Regardless, you must learn proper exercise technique from the beginning. If you've already spent some significant time in the gym you may consider yourself advanced and want to skip right past the technique descriptions that follow. I urge you to reconsider. Even the most seasoned among us can often glean or re-conjure a few morsels that may correct or reorient us back on the optimal path of performance. And the inexperienced would be prudent to heed the sage advice of the masters—

greatness resides in those who spend the time to master the movements, only then adding in the magic elixir of progressive resistance, consistency, determination, heart and intelligence.

From these 80+ exercises, you will be able to follow, and eventually construct workouts that meet your specific goals. Note that you can perform all of these exercises (and the workouts) with a standard free weight barbell, and I encourage you to do so as soon as possible.

If this is your first time performing a specific exercise, go through the motions with the empty bar until the patterning of the movement becomes natural and familiar. Only then, start adding weight. One of the worst mistakes you can make is to prematurely add weight before the correct movement pattern has been established. Bad habits are hard to break.

The second part of this book provides you with lots of workouts for increasing strength and muscle mass, as well as improving weak areas and performing circuit training and cardio work, so you'll be able to put these exercises to use immediately.

One final note regarding each exercise listed—many of the exercises share common tips and techniques for optimum results, so I've repeated those details for each exercise. This provides you with a self-contained reference for each exercise, which I think you'll find especially useful as you continue to use this book as a reference in the future.

Abdominals

You can work abs on the Smith Machine? Well, no. However, you can use the machine itself to set your body in position to work your abs effectively. Read on.

Remember, the purpose of your abdominal muscles is to move your chest towards your waist, flex the spinal column and lift the ribs and move them together (move your waist toward your chest).

Most people are familiar with sit-ups and crunches. You can do those here and the Smith Machine will help put you in position for that. However, most individuals have weakness in their lower abs (bringing their waist towards their chest—not an everyday movement unless you work at the circus or in Las Vegas), which can lead to lower back weakness, general core instability, and all kinds of bad stuff as you move around less and age. The Smith Machine can help you take hold of your efforts to improve your lower abdominal strength and development.

There is a big difference between leg raises and reverse crunches. Leg raises primarily engage your hip flexor muscles, whereas reverse crunches largely remove those muscles from the movement and isolate your abdominal wall. This is why most people who religiously perform leg raises to exclusion wonder why their abdominal strength just isn't up to par. However, just because reverse crunches are so good for you, doesn't mean you should neglect or omit leg raises as well. We all need strong hip flexors to perform basic human movements.

Here are the Smith Machine exercises for the abdominals, in order of increasing effectiveness and difficulty (the more difficult, the more effective and the greater and quicker the results):

- Sit-Ups
- Crunches
- Leg Raises, Hanging, Alternate
- Leg Raises, Hanging, Bent-Knee
- Leg Raises, Hanging, Straight-Leg
- Hanging Reverse Crunches
- Side Bends

Sit-Ups

Works the upper abdominals and hip flexors.

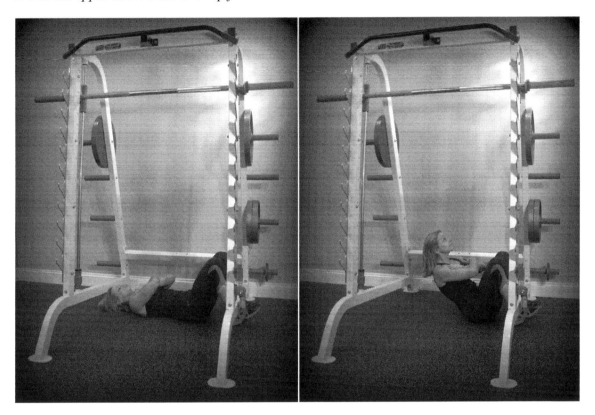

Most people call these sit-ups, but a better visualization term is 'trunk curls'. Think of curling your trunk toward your waist as you sit up.

Performance

Lock the Smith Machine bar at the lowest position. Lie on the floor, bend your knees and hook your feet under the bar or use the machine's armature to secure your feet in the sit-up position. Close your hands into fists and place them at the sides of your head, near your temples—don't place your hands behind your neck; allow the abs to do all the work. Using the strength of your abdominals, curl your body up until your elbows are near your knees. Squeeze your abs and slowly return to the starting position.

Variations

Decline Sit-Ups

If you have difficulty performing standard sit-ups on a flat surface you can set up a declined bench to make this exercise easier. Set up a bench on a decline (use a flat bench with an aerobic step or 45lb plate under one end). Your head and shoulders lie on the inclined section—when you perform the movement, it will be downhill and much easier.

Incline Sit-Ups

Set up a bench on an incline (use a flat bench with an aerobic step or 45lb plate under one end). Your head and shoulders lie on the declined section. Because you are rising uphill from that declined position, this version is more difficult than the standard flat-surface version described above.

Weighted Sit-Ups

Hold a weight plate or dumbbell against your chest (not behind your head!) when performing sit-ups. This allows you to use progressive resistance as your abdominals get stronger.

Twisting Sit-Ups

As you rise up into the full sit-up position, you can turn slightly to the side—this will increase the engagement of your oblique muscles at the sides of your waist. You can alternate turning to each side or perform a single set turning one way, then the subsequent set turning the other. Combine this with the weighted variation above to employ progressive resistance on the oblique muscles.

Tips & Technique

- Sit-up difficulty can be adjusted by changing the surface angle, arm position, and external load you use. Moving from a declined, to flat, to an inclined surface, increases the difficulty. Similarly, and concurrently, you can graduate the difficulty of the exercise via the placement of your arms from your sides, to your chest, to the head, to extension above the head. Holding increasing loads via plates or dumbbells against your chest is the ultimate in progressive resistance sit-up variation. Holding a dumbbell is recommended over a plate, because dumbbells provide smaller incremental load increases.

- Start each rep from the fully reclined position—don't turn this into a partial-range, rapid-fire Sisyphean movement. Abdominals are like any other muscle group, so train them that way.

- Perform a few easy, slow back extensions on the floor after finishing this exercise in order to stretch your abs.

Crunches

Works the upper abdominals.

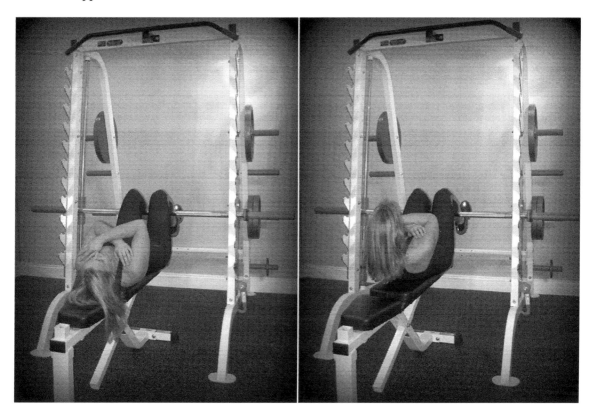

Although sit-ups work both your upper abdominals and hip flexors, crunches allow for more direct isolation of the abdominals while eliminating the hip flexors.

Performance

Lock the Smith Machine bar at a height where your lower legs are parallel to the floor or bench when you are in the proper crunch position. Lie on the floor or a bench, bend your legs until your thighs are perpendicular to the floor and calves are resting on top of the bar. Close your hands into fists and place them at the sides of your head, near your temples—don't place your hands behind your neck; allow the abs to do all the work. Using the strength of your abdominals, try to curl your chest toward your waist. This should bring your shoulders a couple inches off the floor. Hold that position for a second, squeezing your abs hard. Slowly lower to the starting position.

Variations

Decline Crunches

You can use a declined bench to make this exercise easier. Set up a bench on a decline (use a flat bench with an aerobic step or 45lb plate under one end). Your head and shoulders lie on the inclined section—when you perform the movement, it will be downhill and much easier.

Incline Crunches

Set up a bench on an incline (use a flat bench with an aerobic step or 45lb plate under one end). Your head and shoulders lie on the declined section. Because you are rising uphill from that declined position, this version is more difficult than the standard flat-surface version described above.

Weighted Crunches

Hold a weight plate or dumbbell against your chest (not behind your head!) when performing crunches. This allows you to use progressive resistance as your abdominals get stronger.

Twisting Crunches

By turning slightly to the side as you curl into the full crunch position, this will increase the engagement of your oblique muscles at the sides of your waist. You can alternate turning to each side or perform a single set turning one way, then the subsequent set turning the other. Combine this with the weighted variation above to employ progressive resistance on the oblique muscles.

Tips & Technique

- Crunch difficulty can be adjusted by changing the surface angle, arm position, and external load you use. Moving from a declined, to flat, to an inclined surface, increases the difficulty. Similarly, and concurrently, you can graduate the difficulty of the exercise via the placement of your arms from your sides, to your chest, to the head, to extension above the head. Holding increasing loads via plates or dumbbells against your chest is the ultimate in progressive resistance crunch variation. Holding a dumbbell is recommended over a plate, because dumbbells provide smaller incremental load increases.

- Start each rep from the fully reclined position—don't turn this into a partial-range, rapid-fire Sisyphean movement. Abdominals are like any other muscle group, so train them that way.

- Perform a few easy, slow back extensions on the floor after finishing this exercise in order to stretch your abs.

Leg Raises, Hanging, Alternate

Works the lower abs.

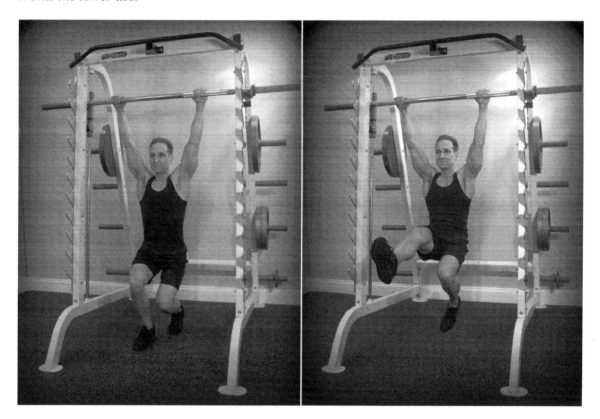

Performance

Lock the bar of the Smith Machine at the highest level available and set the safeties to keep it secured in that position. Hang from the bar using an overhand grip about shoulder width apart. Keeping your legs bent, lift one of your legs out in front of you as high as possible. Slowly lower the leg back down to the starting position and repeat with the other leg.

Tips & Technique

- Gravity works against us most of our lives, so this is a great exercise which coerces gravity into giving us a little payback. Just the act of hanging by our arms helps to stretch out the shoulders, arms, chest, back and spine. If the day has pounded you down, performing hanging exercises will have you standing a little taller and feeling a little better at day's end.

- Because you only need to raise one leg at a time, this version represents the easiest form of this exercise to get started with. Additionally, unilateral movements like this are useful in assessing if you have any strength imbalances between the two sides of the body.

Leg Raises, Hanging, Bent-Knee

Works the lower abs.

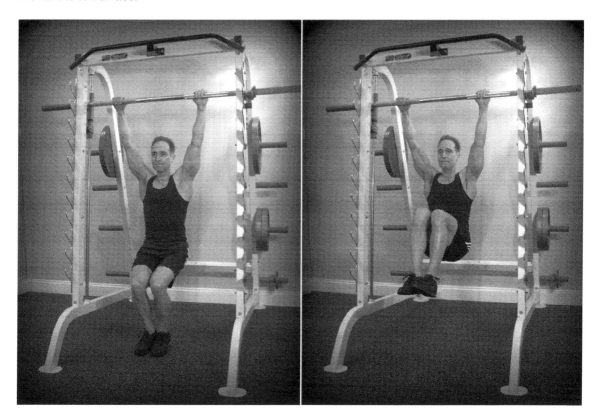

Performance

Lock the bar of the Smith Machine at the highest level available and set the safeties to keep it secured in that position. Hang from the bar using an overhand grip about shoulder width apart. Keeping your legs bent, lift both of them out in front of you as high as possible. Slowly lower the legs back down to the starting position and repeat.

Tips & Technique

- This version of the leg raise is a little more difficult than the single-leg variety because the abs need to lift the entire weight of the lower body.

- Try to hold the contracted position for 1-2 seconds. For a real challenge, try holding that position for up to five seconds between reps. If you have problems with your grip giving out before your abdominals have weakened, consider using a set of wrist straps to hook your hands to the bar.

- To increase the difficulty, you can hold a dumbbell between your feet. This might feel awkward at first, but with a little practice is quickly mastered.

Leg Raises, Hanging, Straight Leg

Works the lower abs.

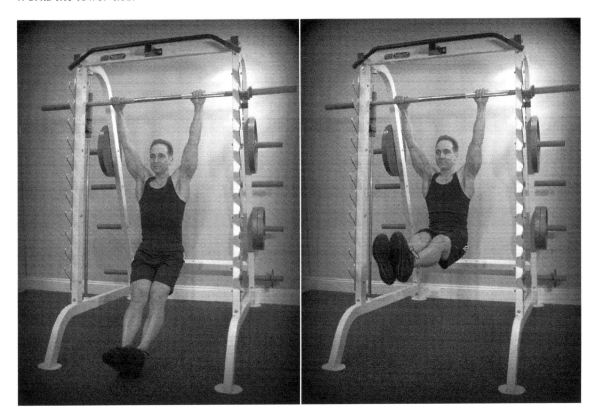

Performance

Lock the bar of the Smith Machine at the highest level available and set the safeties to keep it secured in that position. Hang from the bar using an overhand grip about shoulder width apart. Keeping your legs straight, lift them out in front of you as high as possible. Slowly lower the legs back down to the starting position and repeat.

Tips & Technique

- This is the most difficult version of the leg raise, because simple physics dictate that the further away the weight is from us when we lift it, the heavier the load. Here, the straightened legs provide that distance.

- Try to hold the contracted position for 1-2 seconds. For a real challenge, every once in a while, try holding that position for up to five seconds between reps. If you have problems with your grip giving out before your abdominals have weakened, consider using a set of wrist straps to hook your hands to the bar.

- To increase the difficulty, you can hold a dumbbell between your feet. This might feel awkward at first, but with a little practice is quickly mastered. Because the dumbbell is so far away from you in this variation of the exercise, a light dumbbell quickly presents a serious challenge.

Hanging Reverse Crunches

Works the lower abs.

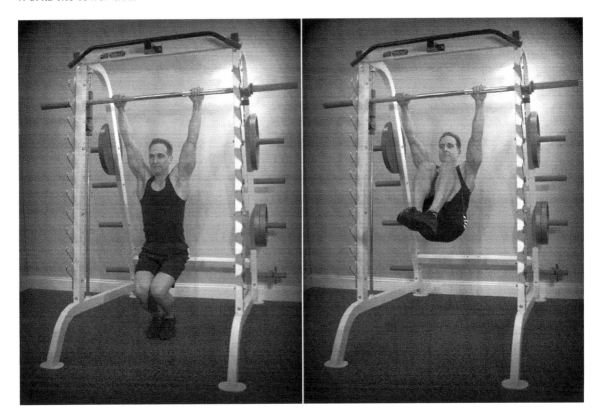

Performance

Lock the bar of the Smith Machine at the highest level available and set the safeties to keep it secured in that position. Hang from the bar using an overhand grip about shoulder width apart. Bend your legs so your thighs are parallel with the floor and your lower legs are pointing to the floor—this is the starting position. Now, here's the hard part. Using only the strength of your abs, try to curl your waist up to your chest. Visualize bringing your knees to your shoulders. Go as high as you can (a few inches for some individuals, a few feet for others). Squeeze your abs hard when you can go no higher, then slowly lower to the starting position. Try not to swing or sway as you perform the reps—you want your abs and not momentum to carry the day here.

Variations

Twisting Reverse Crunches

Turn slightly to the side as you curl your body upward—this will increase the engagement of your oblique muscles at the sides of your waist. You can alternate turning to each side or perform a single set turning one way, then the subsequent set turning the other.

Tips & Technique

- To increase the difficulty, you can hold a dumbbell between your feet. This might feel awkward at first, but with a little practice is quickly mastered.

- For an intensity booster with a unique stress, try squeezing a medicine ball between your knees as you perform this exercise. Not only does this increase the resistance via additional lower body weight, it also activates the muscles of the inner thigh through static contraction. It's like getting two for the price of one and everyone likes a bargain.

- This is near the summit of abdominal exercises in regard to difficulty and effectiveness. Show me someone who can perform a substantial number of reps in this exercise with added weight, and I'll show you someone with exceptional abdominal strength. Master this move and you'll earn your PhD in abdominals—Dr. Abs.

Side Bends

Works the oblique muscles at the sides of your waist.

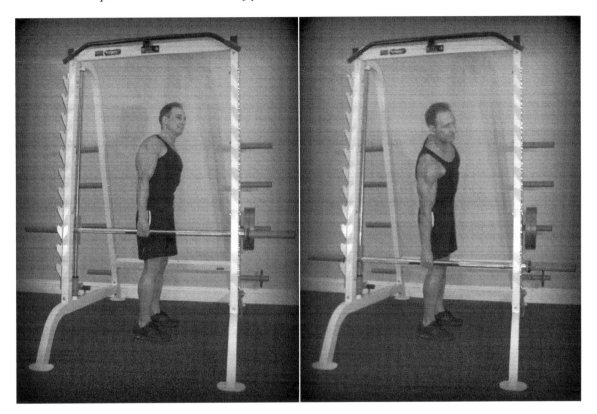

Performance

Lock the bar of the Smith Machine just below knee level. Standing inside of the machine, face toward the side of the machine. Bend your knees so that you can grab the bar with your hand and stand back upright. Keep your legs straight and bend sideways at the waist, lowering the bar as far as possible. Pause, and then slowly return to the upright position. Repeat for as many reps as desired, then turn the other direction and repeat the exercise.

Tips & Technique

▪ To increase intensity, add weight to the bar, but never at the expense of form.

▪ Experiment with both high rep (25-50) and heavier low-rep (6-8) sets in alternating sessions to experience the effect of these extremes. Most of the time, you'll probably find that 15-25 reps work well.

- The oblique muscles are not exempt from the immutable laws of physical change and muscle growth. They are muscles after all, and making them stronger will make them bigger, which equates to occupying more physical space—all other things being equal, your waist will get slightly larger. The key here is to not allow all other things to be equal and strive to reduce your overall body fat. That will make your waist vastly smaller in the end, regardless of your oblique development. In any case, the side bend is a hinge movement and shouldn't be neglected.

- You'll know the next day if these had any effect—like muscle soreness in calves, you can't escape oblique soreness unless you are sleeping.

Back

The purpose of the back musculature is to pull your shoulders down and back—therefore, exercises for the back are all about pulling things, whether it's with a barbell or pulling yourself up to a chinning bar. The Smith Machine makes a good pulling apparatus for various rowing and pull-up motions.

Because the back represents a large collection of interconnected muscles, it responds well to greater volume and variety (exercises, grips, and rep ranges) than other smaller muscle groups. Use this knowledge when constructing your own workouts.

The important concepts in all back exercises include ensuring a full range of motion and visualizing and actualizing pulling your elbows down and back. Don't worry about where your hands are—just think "elbows down and back". If you do that, proper form is quick to follow. Also, try varying your grip width across all rowing and chinning exercises—wide grips tend to emphasize the inner back, whereas narrow grips work the outer back.

Here are the Smith Machine exercises to work your back:

- Bent-Over Rows
- One-Arm Rows
- Incline Bench Rows
- Deadlifts
- Deadlifts, Sumo
- Deadlifts, Partial ("Rack Pulls")
- Good Mornings
- Chins, Behind the Neck, Wide-Grip
- Chins, Close-Grip
- Chins, To the Front
- Pull-Ups
- Inverted Pull-Ups

Bent-Over Rows

Thickens the upper back. Also works the traps and rear shoulders.

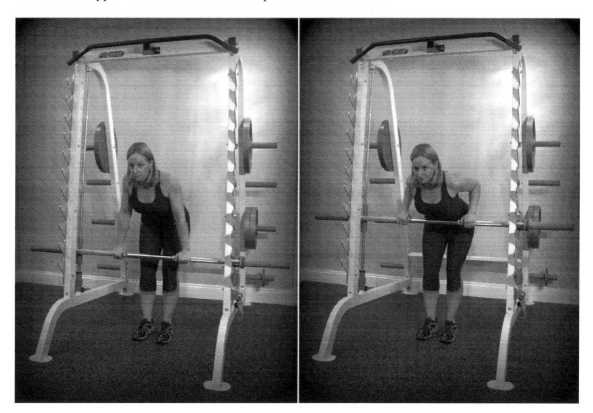

Performance

Set the bar on the Smith Machine to the lowest position (you won't need the safeties for this exercise). Stand with your feet shoulder-width apart. With your knees slightly bent, bend over to hold the bar with a shoulder-width overhand grip. While staying bent at the waist so the body is nearly parallel to the floor and the back is straight, pull the bar to your upper abdominal region and then slowly return to the starting position. It is important to keep the movement controlled and the back straight throughout the exercise. If the Smith Machine does not allow the bar to be lowered far enough, stand on an aerobic step or two plates (one under each foot).

Variations

Reverse-Grip Bent-Over Rows
Instead of holding the bar with an overhand grip, as shown and described above, turn your wrists so

your palms face forward when gripping the bar (reverse grip). Try alternating your grip from workout to workout for maximum benefit.

Wide-Grip Bent-Over Rows

By using a wider than shoulder-width grip, more of the inner back and rear shoulder musculature is affected. Try both overhand and reverse grips for this variation.

Narrow-Grip Bent-Over Rows

By using a narrower than shoulder-width grip, more of the outer back musculature is affected. Try both overhand and reverse grips for this variation.

70-Degree Bent-Over Row

In this variation, bend over and position your straightened back at a 70-degree angle to the floor. That angle should remain constant during the exercise. Additionally, using a reverse-grip with this variation allows you to use more weight and provide additional overload to the back. The stress is shifted more to the mid-back region here.

Tips & Technique

- Keep your upper body position constant throughout the exercise. Resist the temptation to jerk the weight up or use any body movement—pull the bar into your upper abs and squeeze for maximum effectiveness.

- Position your body appropriately, and try pulling the bar to differing destinations—to the navel, the lower chest, the mid-chest or higher. Note the effect that each has on your body. This is useful information, especially when correcting weaknesses later.

- If your lower back is injured, try performing Incline Bench Rows or One-Arm Rows as a substitute, because these exercises provide support for that region.

One-Arm Rows

Isolates each side of the back and really works the lower lats.

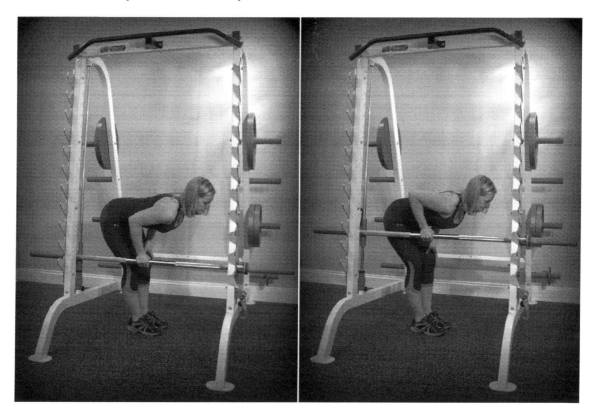

Performance

Set the bar on the Smith Machine to the lowest position (you won't need the safeties for this exercise). You can perform this exercise facing straight ahead (like the **Bent-Over Row**) or by standing sideways in the machine, parallel to the bar (as pictured above). Hold the bar in one hand, and bend forward at the waist until your body is nearly parallel to the floor. With your arm extended to the floor, pull the bar up to your side keeping the elbow in. Lower the bar slowly and repeat. If the Smith Machine does not allow the bar to be lowered far enough, stand on an aerobic step or a barbell plate.

Tips & Technique

▪ Keep your upper body position constant throughout the exercise. Resist the temptation to jerk the weight up or use any body movement—pull the bar into your upper abs and squeeze for maximum effectiveness.

- A common mistake is to slightly rotate your torso away from the bar as you pull it into your ribcage area, using your entire upper torso as leverage for the lift. If you notice this occurring, reduce the weight and re-condition yourself to pull the weight with a steady, uncompromising torso.

- If you have a minor low back injury, try supporting yourself with your non-lifting arm on your thigh (as pictured above).

- This is a great exercise for developing the lower portion of the lats. It's also one of the only unilateral back movements you can perform on a Smith Machine, so take advantage of that. Unilateral movements increase intensity and surface weaker, problematic areas—knowledge that becomes useful for performing corrective actions.

Incline Bench Rows

Isolates and thickens the upper back.

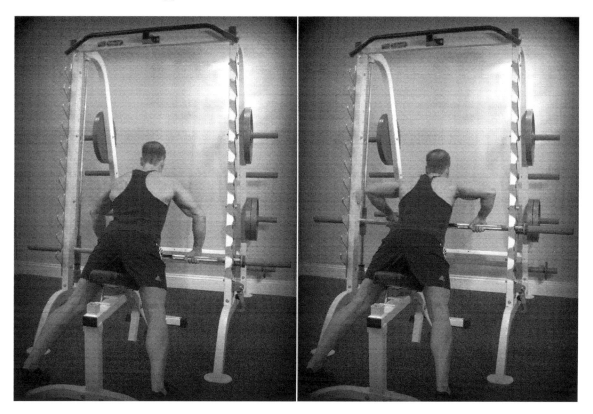

This is an excellent way to perform rows on the Smith Machine when your lower back is fatigued or injured, because your upper body is supported by the bench.

Performance

Set the bar on the Smith Machine to the lowest position. Place an exercise bench, set at a moderate incline (20-40 degrees works well), just in front of or behind the bar. Lie with your chest on the bench, and grab the bar with a shoulder width grip. Without moving your chest up off the bench, pull the weight up in a rowing motion. Squeeze your back at the top of the movement and slowly lower to the starting position.

Variations

Wide-Grip Bench Rows

By using a wider than shoulder-width grip, more of the inner back and rear shoulder musculature is affected.

Narrow-Grip Bench Rows

By using a narrower than shoulder-width grip, more of the outer back musculature is affected.

Tips & Technique

- Try to keep your upper torso in contact with the bench throughout the movement. Resist the temptation to lift your chest off the bench in an effort to lift the weight. Any rising of the torso from the bench activates the spinal erectors of the lower lumbar region of the back. If you are performing this exercise due to a low back issue, lifting your torso away from the bench may nullify that decision.

Deadlifts

Works the entire back, especially the lower back. Also works the glutes, hamstrings and traps.

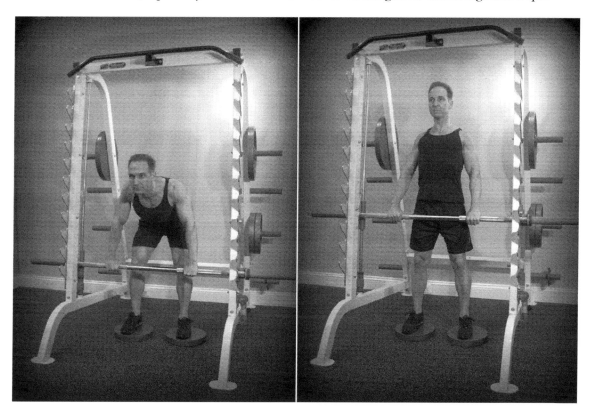

Deadlifts may be the closest thing we have to a universal test of absolute strength. They are a wonderful, superior movement for developing the back.

Performance

Set the bar on the Smith Machine to the lowest position. From a standing position with your shins almost touching the bar, bend your knees slightly and lean forward to grip the bar at shoulder width. Pull the bar upward by extending the hips forward and straightening the legs. Once fully upright, hold this position for a second and then slowly return to the starting position. Remember to keep your back and arms straight, and your shoulders pulled back throughout the exercise.

Tips & Technique

- Throughout the movement, keep your hips low, your arms and back straight and the shoulders back. Failure to keep the back straight can result in injury to the low back.

- Try different stance widths. For many, heels close together with the feet pointing out at 30-degree angles works wonders.

Deadlifts, Sumo

Works the lower back. Also works the hamstrings and traps.

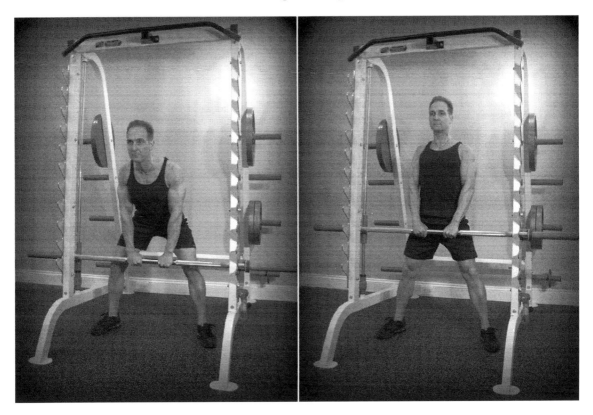

Sumo deadlifts place less stress on your lower back than regular deadlifts. However, they don't work the quadriceps and glutes as hard due to a more limited range of motion, but they do fully engage the hamstrings.

Performance

Set the bar on the Smith Machine to the lowest position. From a standing position with your feet wider than shoulder width and your toes pointing out at 30-degree angles, bend your knees and lean forward to grip the bar. Hold the bar with your hands spaced at shoulder width or narrower, and make sure your arms are straight. Your shins should be vertical. This is the classic starting position for the Sumo Deadlift. Pull the bar to a standing position by extending the hips forward and straightening the legs. Once fully upright, hold this position for a second and then slowly return to the starting position. Remember to keep your back straight throughout the exercise.

Tips & Technique

- Your body should be close to the bar, the shins should be vertical, and your knees should point in the same direction as your feet throughout the exercise. The arms should always be straight, from start to finish.

- If you have relatively short arms, Sumo Deadlifts may be more attuned to your body mechanics than traditional deadlifts.

Deadlifts, Partial ("Rack Pulls")

Works the lower back. Also works the traps and hamstrings.

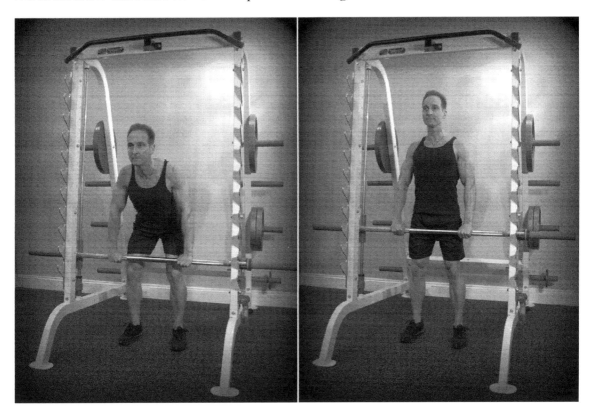

This exercise puts a little less stress on your lower back due to the elevated starting position, while allowing you to use more weight than you can with regular deadlifts.

Performance

Set the bar on the Smith Machine to a position slightly below your knees using the safeties. From a standing position, move your hips backward, bend your knees and lean forward to grab the bar at shoulder width. Pull the bar to a standing position by extending the hips forward and straightening the legs. Once fully upright, hold this position for a second and then slowly return to the starting position. Remember to keep your back straight throughout the exercise.

Tips & Technique

- If you have minor low back issues, this form of partial deadlift, using lighter weights, may assist in rehabbing your back.

- This is also an excellent exercise for overloading the traps, especially when used in conjunction with longer holds (2-3 seconds) at the top of each rep.

Good Mornings

Works the lower back in isolation. Also works the hamstrings.

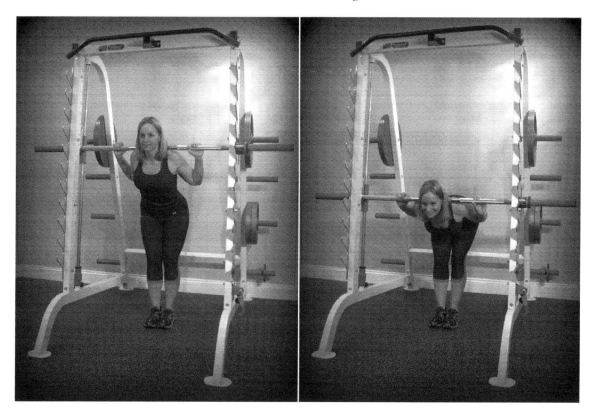

Performance

Set the bar at shoulder height and set the safeties at waist level. Stand with your feet about shoulder width apart, with the bar resting on your upper back behind your neck. Lean forward at the waist until your upper body is parallel to the floor, keeping your knees locked and back straight. Slowly return to the starting position.

Variations

Bent-Knee Good Mornings

For those with less hamstring flexibility, you can bend the knees slightly to compensate for this. Over time, you should be able to move to the standard, straight-leg version of this lift.

Tips & Technique

- It's essential that you start with extremely light weight or no weight if you are new to this exercise.

- Don't perform this exercise if you have a serious low back injury, because it places direct stress on that area.

- For minor low back ailments, perform this exercise using high reps, as described in the **Injury Rehab & Prevention** section.

- Ensure that your back remains straight throughout the exercise. Rounding of the back may cause injury.

- The range of motion you can achieve on this exercise will depend on your degree of flexibility. Don't force the range any lower than a mild stretch. Over time, your flexibility will improve as you work at it.

Chins, Behind the Neck, Wide-Grip

To widen the upper back and create a full sweep in the lats.

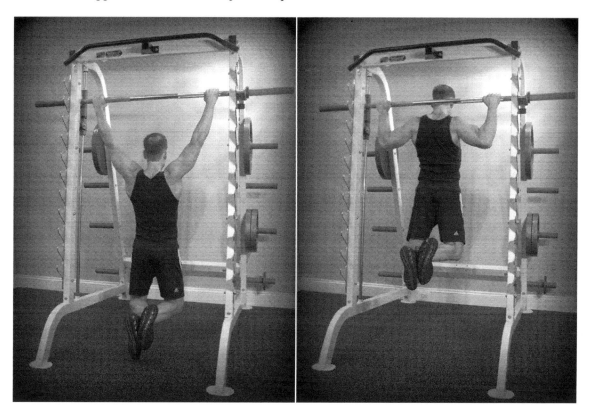

Performance

Lock the bar of the Smith Machine into the topmost position and set the safeties to keep it there. Hang from the bar with an overhand grip keeping the arms wider than shoulder width. Pull yourself up so that your head rises above the height of the bar. Slowly return to the starting position and repeat.

Variations

Weighted Chins, Behind the Neck
Once you can perform at least three sets of twelve reps with your body weight on this exercise, you may want to consider using a dipping belt or holding a dumbbell between the feet to provide additional resistance.

Tips & Technique

- The most common mistake in any chinning or pull-up exercise is failure to use a full range of motion. As you probably learned in school gym class, you start by hanging from the bar with straight arms and your chin/head should be able to clear the bar at the top of the movement. That's the correct way. The first point is easy to confirm—ensure that you start *each rep* from a dead hang position. If your arms are even slightly bent, that's wrong. Second, if you can't pull yourself up to clear your chin or head over the bar then use the **Inverted Pull-Ups** exercise and slowly increase the height of the bar as you get stronger. Failure to use a full range of motion on this exercise only cheats yourself, your ultimate development of strength and muscle in the back region and attainment of the classic Greek V-taper from upper back to the waist. Yes, it's a pride-swallowing moment to re-pattern this movement if you've been fooling yourself over the years, but if you truly want optimal results, acting on truth and honesty always leads you in the direction of the promised land. Over time, this exercise will make your waist appear smaller.

- Don't neglect the lowering portion of the movement. This eccentric lowering action should always be performed under control for both safety and maximum muscle fiber stimulation. In general, the pull to the top of the movement should be relatively quick, whereas the lowering action should be slow and under control at all times.

- One technique you can use to gradually empower and strengthen yourself for performing a full rep on chins is to stand on an exercise bench to get yourself into the fully contracted position (head above the bar). From there, lift your feet from the bench and slowly lower yourself to a dead hang position, resisting gravity as much as possible on the way down. These are called negative reps. The longer it takes you to lower yourself, the stronger you are getting. For the truly strong, you can use this same technique with a dipping belt and attached weights to lower yourself and some titanic poundage back to terra firma.

Chins, Close-Grip

To widen the lower lats and develop the serratus.

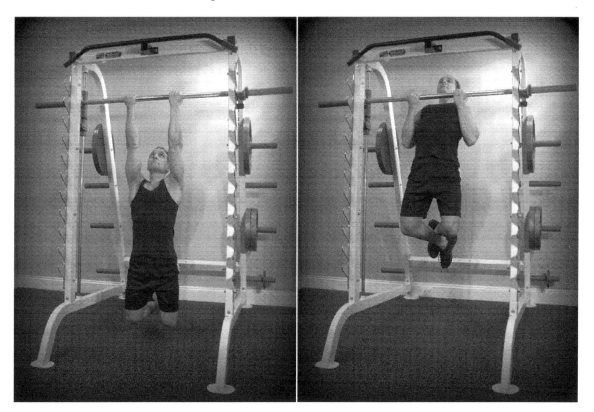

Performance

Lock the bar of the Smith Machine into the topmost position and set the safeties to keep it there. Hang from the bar with your hands close together—about shoulder width or slightly narrower. Pull yourself up leaning your head back while attempting to touch your chest to the bar at the top of the movement. Slowly return to the starting position.

Tips & Technique

- This exercise also helps develop the serratus muscles—these are the small, finger-like muscles at the sides of your rib cage, visible when you look into a mirror with your arms extended overhead. If you can't see them, it's either because they aren't sufficiently developed or your body fat level is obscuring them.

- The most common mistake in any chinning or pull-up exercise is failure to use a full range of motion. As you probably learned in school gym class, you start by hanging from the bar with straight arms and your chin/head should be able to clear the bar at the top of the movement. That's the correct way. The first point is easy to confirm—ensure that you start *each rep* from a dead hang position. If your arms are even slightly bent, that's wrong. Second, if you can't pull yourself up to clear your chin or head over the bar then use the Inverted Pull-Ups exercise and slowly increase the height of the bar as you get stronger. Failure to use a full range of motion on this exercise only cheats yourself, your ultimate development of strength and muscle in the back region and attainment of the classic Greek V-taper from upper back to the waist. Yes, it's a pride-swallowing moment to re-pattern this movement if you've been fooling yourself over the years, but if you truly want optimal results, acting on truth and honesty always leads you in the direction of the promised land. Over time, this exercise will make your waist appear smaller.

- Don't neglect the lowering portion of the movement. This eccentric lowering action should always be performed under control for both safety and maximum muscle fiber stimulation. In general, the pull to the top of the movement should be relatively quick, whereas the lowering action should be slow and under control at all times.

- One technique you can use to gradually empower and strengthen yourself to performing a full rep on chins is to stand on an exercise bench to get yourself into the fully contracted position (head above the bar). From there, slowly lower yourself to a dead hang position, resisting gravity as much as possible on the way down. These are called negative reps. The longer it takes you to lower yourself, the stronger you are getting. For the truly strong, you can use this same technique with a dipping belt and attached weights to lower yourself and some titanic poundage back to terra firma.

Chins, To the Front

To widen the upper back and create a full sweep in the lats.

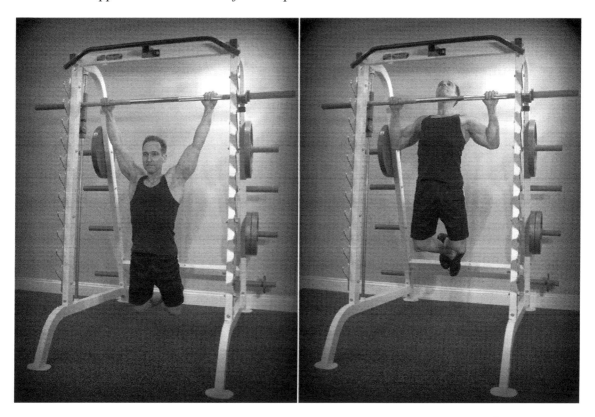

Performance

Lock the bar of the Smith Machine into the topmost position and set the safeties to keep it there. Hang from the bar with an overhand grip keeping your arms at shoulder width or slightly wider. Pull yourself up so that the top of your chest touches the bar (great) or your head rises above the bar (good). Slowly return to the starting position and repeat.

Tips & Technique

▪ It's good to alternate chinning to the front and to the rear either within or across workouts. Although both work the latissimus muscles of the back, the purely vertical rear chins tend to help etch the detail into the upper back across the shoulder blades—you're pulling straight down. With front chins, the pull is down and slightly back.

- The most common mistake in any chinning or pull-up exercise is failure to use a full range of motion. As you probably learned in school gym class, you start by hanging from the bar with straight arms and your chin/head should be able to clear the bar at the top of the movement. That's the correct way. The first point is easy to confirm—ensure that you start *each rep* from a dead hang position. If your arms are even slightly bent, that's wrong. Second, if you can't pull yourself up to clear your chin or head over the bar then use the **Inverted Pull-Ups** exercise and slowly increase the height of the bar as you get stronger. Failure to use a full range of motion on this exercise only cheats yourself, your ultimate development of strength and muscle in the back region and attainment of the classic Greek V-taper from upper back to the waist. Yes, it's a pride-swallowing moment to re-pattern this movement if you've been fooling yourself over the years, but if you truly want optimal results, acting on truth and honesty always leads you in the direction of the promised land. Over time, this exercise will make your waist appear smaller.

- Don't neglect the lowering portion of the movement. This eccentric lowering action should always be performed under control for both safety and maximum muscle fiber stimulation. In general, the pull to the top of the movement should be relatively quick, whereas the lowering action should be slow and under control at all times.

- One technique you can use to gradually empower and strengthen yourself to performing a full rep on chins is to stand on an exercise bench to get yourself into the fully contracted position (head above the bar). From there, slowly lower yourself to a dead hang position, resisting gravity as much as possible on the way down. These are called negative reps. The longer it takes you to lower yourself, the stronger you are getting. For the truly strong, you can use this same technique with a dipping belt and attached weights to lower yourself and some titanic poundage back to terra firma.

Pull-Ups

Thickens the upper back. Also works the biceps.

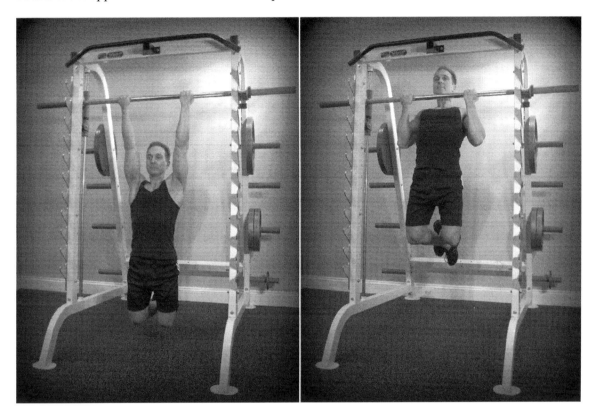

This is the standard pull-up you probably learned in school. Along with reading, writing and arithmetic, it is a basic skill that everyone should have.

Performance

Lock the bar of the Smith Machine into the topmost position and set the safeties to keep it there. Hang from the bar with an underhand grip (palms facing you) keeping your arms about shoulder width apart. Pull yourself up so that the top of your chest touches the bar (great) or your head rises above the bar (good). Slowly return to the starting position and repeat.

Tips & Technique

- Because this exercise uses your biceps, in addition to your lats, to assist in the pulling motion, you should be slightly stronger in this movement than the standard Chins To the Front.

- The most common mistake in any chinning or pull-up exercise is failure to use a full range of motion. As you probably learned in school gym class, you start by hanging from the bar with straight arms and your chin/head should be able to clear the bar at the top of the movement. That's the correct way. The first point is easy to confirm—ensure that you start *each rep* from a dead hang position. If your arms are even slightly bent, that's wrong. Second, if you can't pull yourself up to clear your chin or head over the bar then use the Inverted Pull-Ups exercise and slowly increase the height of the bar as you get stronger. Failure to use a full range of motion on this exercise only cheats yourself, your ultimate development of strength and muscle in the back region and attainment of the classic Greek V-taper from upper back to the waist. Yes, it's a pride-swallowing moment to re-pattern this movement if you've been fooling yourself over the years, but if you truly want optimal results, acting on truth and honesty always leads you in the direction of the promised land. Over time, this exercise will make your waist appear smaller.

- Don't neglect the lowering portion of the movement. This eccentric lowering action should always be performed under control for both safety and maximum muscle fiber stimulation. In general, the pull to the top of the movement should be relatively quick, whereas the lowering action should be slow and under control at all times.

- One technique you can use to gradually empower and strengthen yourself to performing a full rep on chins is to stand on an exercise bench to get yourself into the fully contracted position (head above the bar). From there, slowly lower yourself to a dead hang position, resisting gravity as much as possible on the way down. These are called negative reps. The longer it takes you to lower yourself, the stronger you are getting. For the truly strong, you can use this same technique with a dipping belt and attached weights to lower yourself and some titanic poundage back to terra firma.

Inverted Pull-Ups/Rows

Thickens the upper back.

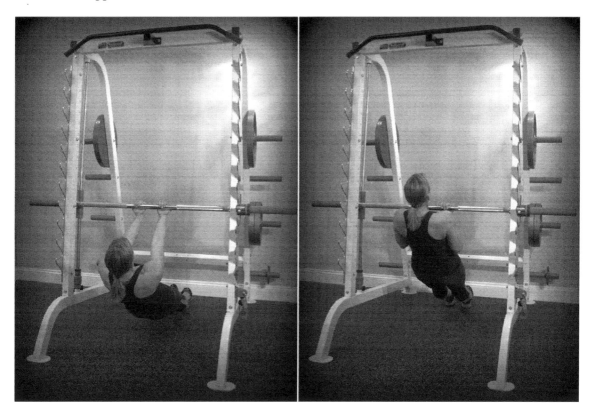

This exercise assists those who have difficulty performing pull-ups with their entire body weight. It's also good when you have fatigued your back from regular pull-ups and want to continue with more, because all you need to do is lower the bar.

Performance

Set the bar of the Smith Machine at about waist height and set the safeties to keep it there. Starting from a lying position on the floor, reach up and grab the bar with an underhand grip keeping your hands at shoulder width or narrower. Pull yourself up so that the top of your chest touches the bar. Your heels should remain on the floor at all times. Slowly return to the starting position and repeat.

Variations

Feet Elevated

By placing the backs of your heels on an elevated surface, such as an exercise bench, you increase the intensity of the exercise.

Tips & Technique

- Make sure the bar is set minimally at a height that allows you to fully extend your arms from the start position.

- As you get stronger in this exercise slowly lock the bar into higher positions along the rails. This increases the resistance. Eventually, you'll be able to perform standard pull-ups. Keep a written record of the position setting you used.

- If you are performing this exercise as a substitute for Bent-Over Rows, bring your stomach up to the bar, instead of your chest. This turns the exercise into an inverted row and shifts the emphasis from the latissimus muscles to the entire back musculature.

- You can also grip the bar with your palms facing away from you. This decreases the involvement of the biceps and makes the exercise more difficult.

- Wider than shoulder-width grips work more of the inner back and rear shoulder musculature, whereas narrower grips affect more of the outer back. Try alternating between various grip widths for complete back development.

Biceps

Ever since "show me your muscles" was first uttered (somewhere in a cave?), arms have been flexing worldwide. Hopefully, you were able to produce at least a small bump on your upper arm on the bus to school that fateful day. This event has led millions of (mostly) men to start lifting weights, setting in motion a sequence of events leading to the gym, the gym in the basement or the athletic field. Hopefully, you are still there and still trying to build those glorious biceps.

Because underhand chin-ups are one of the most basic biceps builders of all time, the Smith Machine will be happy to oblige you here. Before the ancient Greeks invented the precursor to the modern dumbbell (the 'haltere'), man was pulling himself up tree limbs with an underhand grip. Look at any Olympic male gymnast—not a lot of leg mass there, but look at those biceps. What movements do they perform consistently? How about pulling themselves up while holding onto a bar or rings—with an underhand grip.

Additionally, the Smith Machine will allow you to do a few simulated curling variations, if you are in a pinch and don't have access to a barbell or dumbbells.

Before we look at the full array of biceps exercises available, here are some general tips when working this relatively small muscle:

• The biggest mistake that almost all weight trainers make when working biceps is using a limited range of motion. Doing that is like putting a restrictor plate on a racecar. Other common mistakes include using too much weight (right, guys?), using momentum to throw the weight up instead of actually lifting it, and letting your ego dictate your biceps workout. They are all inter-related.

• Stretch your biceps between each set. I can't say this enough. Try a biceps workout without stretching them and another with stretching. Notice the difference?

Here are the Smith Machine exercises to work your biceps:

- Close-Grip Pull-Ups
- Inverted Close-Grip Pull-Ups
- Curls
- Drag Curls
- Reverse Curls

Close-Grip Pull-Ups

Builds overall mass in the biceps.

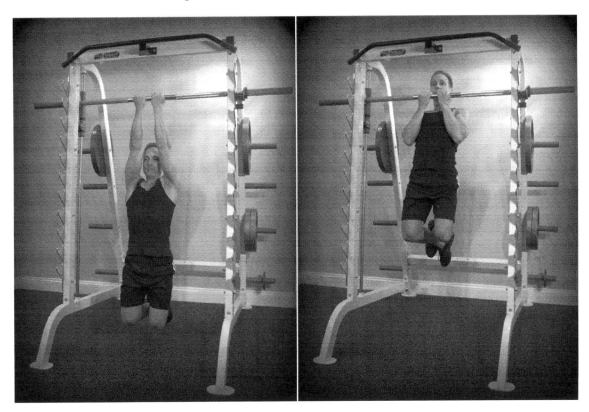

Performance

Lock the bar of the Smith Machine into the topmost position and set the safeties to keep it there. Hang from the bar with your palms facing you and your hands set close together. Slowly pull yourself up, concentrating on using only your biceps. Squeeze your biceps hard at the top and slowly lower yourself until your arms are straight.

Variations

Weighted Close-Grip Pull-Ups
Once you can perform at least three sets of twelve reps with your body weight on this exercise, you may want to consider using a dipping belt or holding a dumbbell between the feet to provide additional resistance.

Tips & Technique

- If you are tall or the Smith Machine is short (such as a home unit), you will probably need to keep your legs bent throughout the movement so they don't touch the floor.

- If you aren't strong enough (yet) for this exercise, substitute the inverted version, described next.

- Don't allow your torso to swing! This will require practice, but make a conscious effort to keep your torso as stable as possible. Concentrate on letting your biceps do the work.

- Don't stop short of full extension—let yourself hang all the way down between each rep and pause at the bottom. This will build bigger and stronger biceps over time. Let all your half-assed friends perform these with partial reps—like the hare and tortoise fable, you'll have the last laugh in the end.

Inverted Close-Grip Pull-Ups

Builds mass in the biceps.

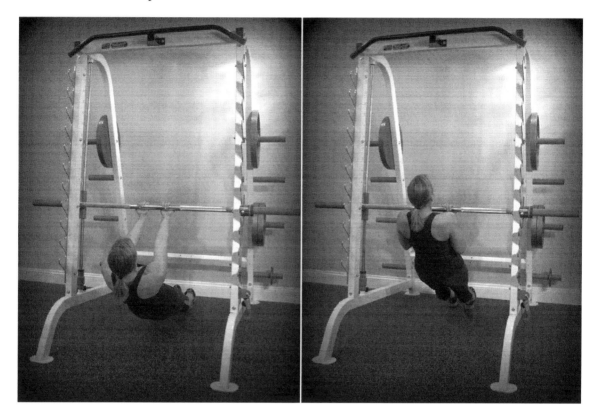

This exercise is useful for those who have trouble doing close-grip pull-ups using their entire body weight.

Performance

Set the bar of the Smith Machine at about waist height and set the safeties to keep it there. Starting from a lying position on the floor, reach up and grab the bar with an underhand grip keeping your hands close together. Slowly pull yourself up, concentrating on using only your biceps. Squeeze your biceps hard at the top and slowly lower until your arms are straight.

Variations

Feet Elevated

By placing the backs of your heels on an elevated surface, such as an exercise bench, you increase the intensity of the exercise.

Neutral-Grip

If you position yourself under the bar, facing sideways in the machine so the bar is in line with your body (your feet may need to extend outside one side of the machine), you can use a close-grip with the palms of your hands facing each other (like you would hold a baseball bat). This provides a hammer-type curl simulation and works the forearm muscles (forearm extensors), as well as some additional bicep muscles (brachialis).

Tips & Technique

- Make sure the bar is set minimally at a height that allows you to fully extend your arms.

- Keep your body straight and rigid throughout the movement. This also helps work your core muscles.

- Eventually, as you get stronger at this exercise slowly lock the bar into higher positions along the rails. This increases the resistance. Eventually, you'll be able to perform standard close-grip pull-ups. Keep a record of the position setting you used.

- The biceps are composed of two main parts—an inner and outer head. The closer the grip width, the more the outer biceps head is stressed. Conversely, the wider the grip, the more the inner head is stressed. Because change is good, make sure to rotate grip widths every other workout for best results.

Curls

Develops the biceps.

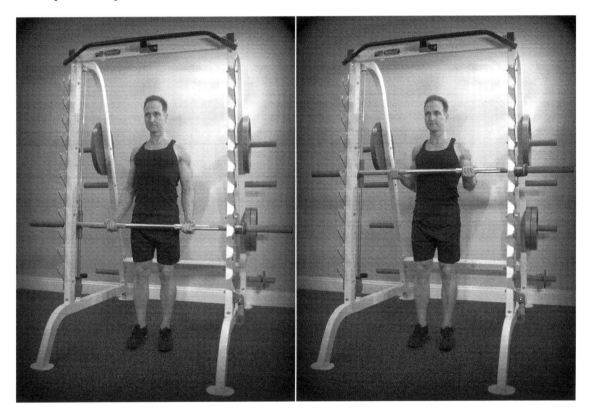

Performance

Set the bar of the Smith Machine at about mid-thigh and set the safeties to keep it there. Unlock and hold the bar using an underhand grip about shoulder width apart. Your body should be about six inches behind the bar. Lift the bar upwards, keeping your elbows close to your sides, until the bar reaches chest level. Slowly return to the starting position and repeat.

Variations

Close-Grip and *Wide-Grip*

The closer the grip width, the more the outer biceps head is stressed. Conversely, the wider the grip, the more the inner head is stressed. It's useful to change your grip width frequently, either within an exercise session or across workouts.

Tips & Technique

- Ensure that you lower the bar as far as possible. Because the Smith Machine is a limiting device in this movement, any further self-imposed limitations on your range of motion limit your results.

- Try holding the contracted position at the top for 1-2 seconds to pattern the finishing portion of the movement. The Smith Machine makes for an effective curl apparatus when slow, controlled movements with linear resistance are desired.

Drag Curls

Develops the biceps.

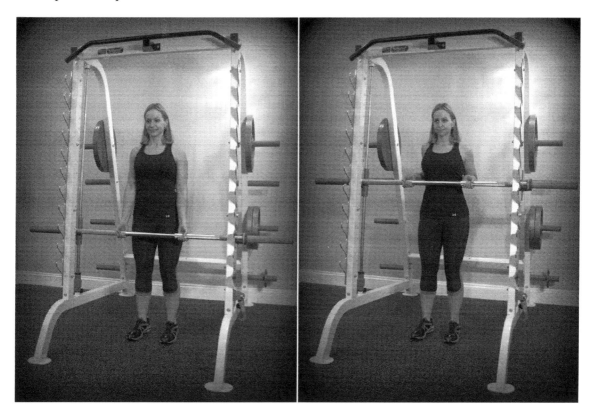

This exercise differs slightly from the standard curl in that it produces a little more of a concentration curl type of simulated movement.

Performance

Set the bar of the Smith Machine at about mid-thigh and set the safeties to keep it there. Unlock and hold the bar using an underhand grip about shoulder width apart. Your body should be almost against the bar. Pull your elbows back and raise the bar to your lower chest, keeping the bar in close contact with your torso. The motion will resemble dragging the bar up the front of your body. Slowly return to the starting position and repeat.

Variations

Close-Grip and *Wide-Grip*

The closer the grip width, the more the outer biceps head is stressed. Conversely, the wider the grip, the more the inner head is stressed. It's useful to change your grip width frequently, either within an exercise session or across workouts.

Tips & Technique

- Because drag curls in any form (barbell, dumbbell, cable) use a linear dragging motion straight up the front of the body, the Smith Machine is well-suited for this exercise.

- The range of motion here is shorter than with standard curls so you might not be able to use as much weight, but don't sacrifice any of that range for additional weight. It's better to control the drag of the bar all the way up to your lower chest and squeeze hard, than to yank up a little more weight than you are really capable of.

Reverse Curls

Develops the outside head of the biceps and the forearm extensors.

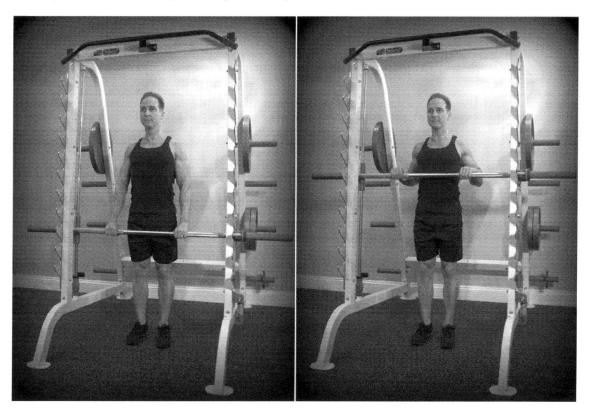

I like to call reverse curls the exercise that time forgot. Weight lifters of the 1950s always performed this movement, and no surprise, they all seemed to have huge forearms and thick biceps.

Performance

While standing, hold the bar with an overhand grip about shoulder width apart. With the bar hanging down in front of you, lift the bar upwards, keeping your elbows close to your sides, until the bar reaches chest level. Slowly return to the starting position and repeat.

Tips & Technique

- Resist the temptation to lean back and pull the bar upward when things get difficult. The brachialis (outside part of the biceps) is a relatively small muscle, so make it do the work in order to reap the rewards. For ultimate results, keep those elbows as close to the body as possible.

- Try varying your grip width and find a width that allows your wrists to co-exist peacefully with this exercise. More often than not, it will be shoulder width or slightly wider.

Calves

You can often thank or curse your parents for the initial state of your calf development. Genetics dictates a large role in calf development, maybe more so than any other muscle group. You've seen them—guys or gals, small and petite with outrageously sized calves, or professional basketball players who consistently perform explosive jumping movements with relatively tiny calves. That's genetics laid bare for all to see.

However, like most things in life, there is a direct correlation between achieving your own calf potential and the workload/effort you put into them. Most don't—so dare to be different.

Although your calves simply flex your foot, here are the important points you need to remember for working them effectively:

- Range of motion is essential with calf work—maybe more so than with any other muscle group. That's because when you walk you work your calves, but only through a partial, middle-ground range of motion. Make your calves work through the other two extremes (full stretch and full contraction) and that's where they really start to respond.

- For complete calf development you also need to work them with both your legs bent (seated) and with them straight (standing), because there are two distinct muscle groups that compose your calves—one of which (the gastrocnemius) is attached above the back of your knee (therefore you must pre-stretch that muscle by keeping your legs straight). The other (the soleus) is attached below the back of your knee and is worked most effectively when your leg is bent.

- Perform your calf exercises with varying foot stance widths. Because the gastrocnemius is composed of two parts (an inner and outer head, much like the biceps), stances wider than shoulder width tend to shift the workload to your inner calf, whereas narrow stances shift it to the outer calf. Try this little experiment right now. Stand in bare feet with your feet placed wider than shoulder width. Keeping your legs completely straight, rise all the way up onto your toes. Notice how most of your weight shifts onto your big toes? The stress is also shifting onto the inner head of the gastrocnemius. Now place your feet together and try it again. Your weight just shifted onto your little toes and the outer head of the gastrocnemius.

- Calves get indirect work when performing squats and deadlifts. The heavier you go in those exercises, the bigger your calves will get. Remember, the body is a unit.

Here are the Smith Machine exercises to work your calves:

- Calf Raises
- Calf Raises, One-Leg
- Calf Raises, Squatting
- Donkey Calf Raises
- Seated Calf Raises
- Tibialis Raises

Calf Raises

Develops the calf muscles.

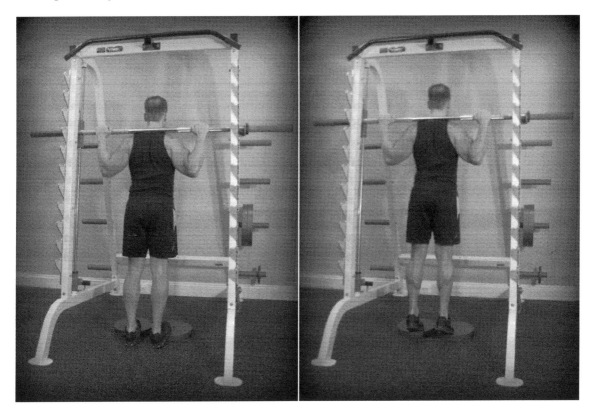

Performance

Place an aerobic step or two 25lb plates on the floor directly under the Smith Machine bar. Place the bar across your upper back and your toes on the step/plates. You should be standing straight up, not leaning forward or back. With your legs straight, rise up as high as you can onto your toes. Slowly lower back down until your heels touch the floor.

Tips & Technique

▪ If you have a sturdy, adjustable aerobic step available, try using that in order to get a greater range of motion and stretch when lowering your heels. Don't stack plates to achieve this—that's dangerous and eventually those plates will shift on you and you'll be looking for the injury rehab section next.

- It's essential to keep your legs straight during this exercise to get maximum results. Don't sacrifice form for weight.

- Try holding the top contracted position for 1-2 seconds before lowering and pause at the bottom of the movement—no bouncing here, unless you want to find out why they call it the Achilles tendon.

Calf Raises, One-Leg

Isolates each set of calf muscles.

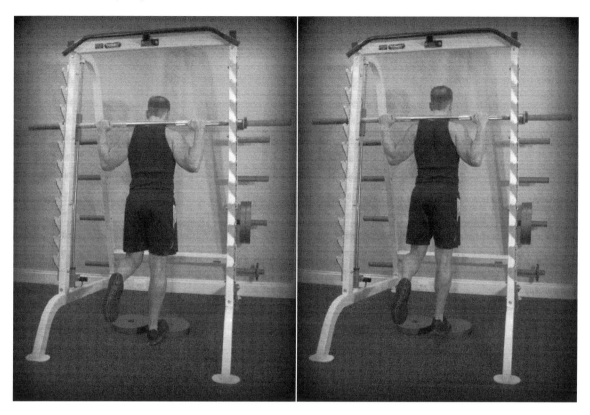

Performing calf raises unilaterally, one leg at a time increases the intensity of the exercise and helps to uncover any muscle imbalances.

Performance

Place an aerobic step or two 25lb plates on the floor directly under the Smith Machine bar. Place the bar across your upper back and your toes on the plates. You should be standing straight up, not leaning forward or back. Keeping one of your legs straight, the other bent backwards, rise up as high as you can onto your toes. Slowly lower back down until your heel touches the floor. Repeat for as many reps as possible, and then switch to the other leg and repeat the process.

Tips & Technique

- If you have a sturdy, adjustable aerobic step available, try using that in order to get a greater range of motion and stretch when lowering your heels. Don't stack plates to achieve this—

that's dangerous, and eventually those plates will shift on you and you'll be looking for the injury rehab section next.

- It's essential to keep your legs straight during this exercise to get maximum results. Don't sacrifice form for weight.

- Try holding the top contracted position for 1-2 seconds before lowering and pause at the bottom of the movement—no bouncing here, especially because your lower tendons were not dipped into the river Styx either, much like Achilles.

- When one calf begins to tire so that you cannot complete a full rep, try using a little assistance from the other calf to reach the top position, then use just the target calf to slowly lower yourself, resisting as much as possible. This negative or eccentric-only movement provides additional intensity and overload to the calf.

- This is a great exercise for discovering, verifying and correcting imbalances between the strength and development of each calf. For many, it's an eye-opener.

Calf Raises, Squatting

Works the calves, especially the soleus.

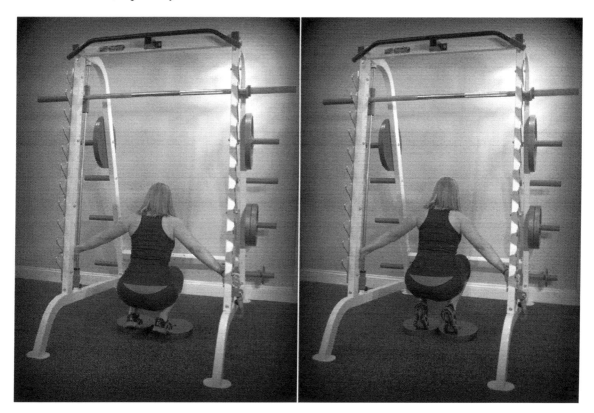

Performance

Set the bar of the Smith Machine at about waist height and set the safeties to keep it there. (Optionally, you can just move the bar to the top position to move it out of the way.) Place an aerobic step or two 25lb plates on the floor directly under the Smith Machine bar. Holding onto the bar or sides of the machine for balance, place your feet close together, the toes of each foot on each plate (or the step), and squat down as far as you can. While remaining in the squatting position, rise up on your toes as high as you can, squeeze your calves hard, then slowly lower until your heels touch the floor. Use only your calves to raise your body—don't use your thighs. Try performing this exercise for extremely high repetitions, such as 50-100.

Variations

One-Leg Squatting Calf Raises
Try performing this exercise with one calf at a time. This will significantly increase both the load and intensity.

Weighted Squatting Calf Raises
If you have a weight vest or backpack, you can wear that to provide additional resistance.

Tips & Technique

- This is a great exercise to use immediately after a set of standing calf raises—you'll be able to hit both primary muscle groups in your calves (gastrocnemius and soleus) in quick fashion.

- The only safe method for increasing the load on this exercise is to strap on a sturdy backpack loaded with plates or by using a weight vest. Combine this with the one-leg variation described above for the ultimate method of performing this exercise.

- Try holding the top contracted position for 1-2 seconds before lowering. Again, no bouncing at the bottom.

Donkey Calf Raises

Develops the thickness of the back of the calves.

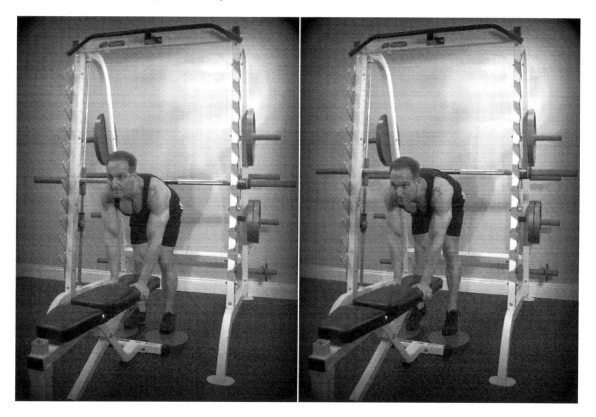

Performance

Place an exercise bench just forward of the Smith Machine. Place two 25lb plates on the floor directly under the Smith Machine bar. Set the bar of the Smith Machine just below waist height and set the safeties to keep it there. Now, place your toes on the 25lb plates, bend over at the waist, hold onto the bench and lift your hips up until the bar rests on your lower back and is not hooked into the machine. Your torso should be approximately parallel to the floor. Start by rising up on your toes as high as possible, squeeze your calves, and then slowly lower until your heels touch the floor. When you are finished performing the exercise, bend your legs to lower the bar back onto the safeties.

Variations

One-Leg Donkey Calf Raises
If you are strong enough, try performing this exercise with one calf at a time. This will significantly increase both the load and intensity.

Tips & Technique

- Although initially somewhat difficult to set up and execute correctly, the payoffs here can be huge. The Donkey Calf Raise is probably the most effective exercise for the gastrocnemius, due to the extreme range of motion involved. Start with an empty or lightly loaded bar and practice the movement.

- Try holding the top contracted position for 1-2 seconds before lowering.

Seated Calf Raises

Develops the lower and outer areas of the calves.

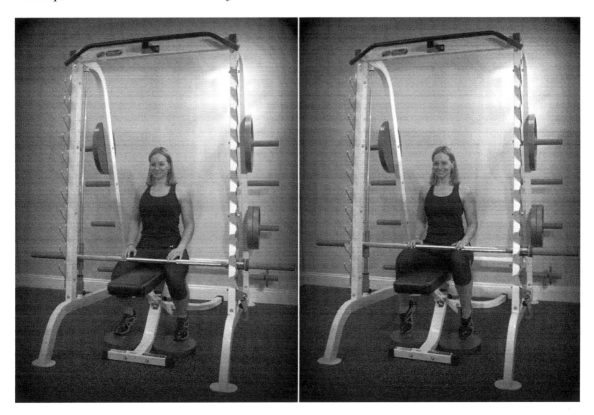

Performance

Place a flat exercise bench directly under the Smith Machine bar. Put a towel around the middle of the bar for padding. Place two 25lb plates on the floor directly to each side of the bench. Lift the bar and sit on the bench with the bar resting across your lower thighs. Place your toes on the 25lb plates. Rise up on your toes as high as possible, hold for a second, and then lower your heels to the floor.

Variations

One-Leg Seated Calf Raises

If you are strong enough, try performing this exercise with one calf at a time. This will significantly increase both the load and intensity.

Tips & Technique

- Ensure that your shins are perpendicular to the floor throughout the movement. They shouldn't be angled forward or back—straight up and down is what you want for maximum stress on the soleus muscle of the calf.

- Try holding the top contracted position for 1-2 seconds before lowering.

Tibialis Raises

Develops the front of the calves.

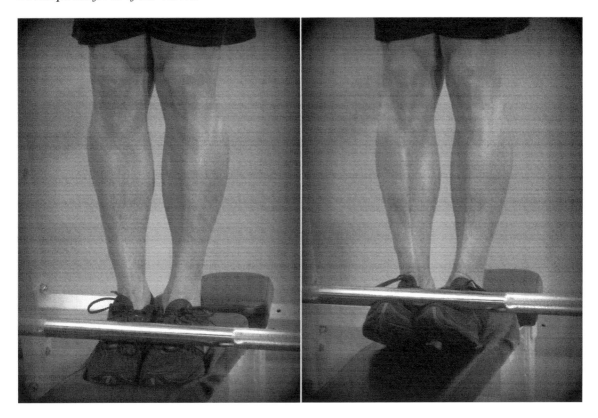

Most people forget (or don't realize) there is a calf muscle in front of your lower leg—the tibialis. This exercise works that area. For some people who get shin splints when jogging or running, this exercise may help alleviate that problem.

Performance

Place a flat exercise bench directly under the Smith Machine bar. Lower the bar until it is resting on the bench. Stand on the bench, lift the bar slightly, place the front of your feet under the bar, and then slowly rest the bar back down on top of your feet. While holding onto the Smith Machine for support, try to lift your toes (and the bar) upward. Pause at the top of the movement, and then slowly lower to the starting position.

Variations

One-Leg Tibialis Raises

If you are strong enough, try performing this exercise with one leg at a time. This will significantly increase both the load and intensity.

Tips & Technique

- This exercise has a limited range of motion because you can't flex your foot upward as far as you can downward. Again, this isn't a movement anyone routinely performs with resistance in daily life, so the key is to use the magic elixir of consistency and progressive resistance to transform this area.

- Try holding the top contracted position for 1-2 seconds before lowering.

Chest

For men, chest is undoubtedly, along with biceps, the most popular and frequently worked muscle group. Unfortunately, for men it's where egos reign and chest development suffers. Women seem to be smarter here.

Horizontal pushing is one of the basic human movements. The Smith Machine will allow you to build and shape your chest by using a variety of pushing movements and hand positions. Although science tells us that you can't work portions of the chest in isolation through pressing movements, bodybuilding practitioners over the past century tend to prove otherwise. Pressing from a flat surface allows you to work the entire chest directly. Incline presses or presses where the bar lowers near the neck shifts part of the stress onto the upper chest (pectorals) and front of the shoulders, enhancing the development of those areas. Decline presses largely remove the upper pectorals from the movement and shift the majority of the stress toward the lower chest.

Here are some other important points for working your chest effectively:

- Don't let your ego pick the weight you use or dictate your form—don't use excessive arch in your back to press the weight up—that just shifts the work to your shoulders. Proper form will build a complete chest more effectively than sloppy form with lots of weight. And your shoulders will be able to function properly decades from now.

- Keep your shoulders pinned back and down on all chest pressing movements. Imagine you are trying to squeeze a marble between your shoulder blades. Set yourself in that position before unlocking the bar and maintain that tightness throughout the movement to maximize pectoral involvement. Think "shoulders back and down" when pressing for the chest.

- Stretch your chest between sets by holding onto the uprights of the Smith Machine and leaning forward until you feel your chest stretch. Remember, the body is a unit and that which pushes must be pulled apart just as often.

Here are the Smith Machine exercises to work your chest:

- Bench Press
- Guillotine Press
- Incline Press
- Decline Press
- Floor Press
- Push Up

Bench Press

Builds mass and strengthens the chest, shoulders and arms.

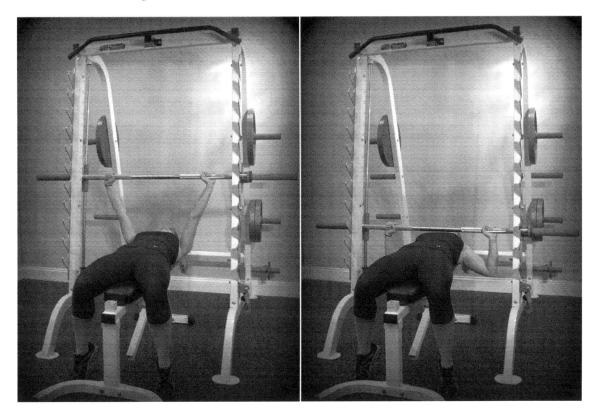

Performance

Place a flat bench under the Smith Machine bar. Set the safeties just above the height of the bench. Lie on the bench, grab the bar with a shoulder width (or slightly wider) grip and unhook the bar. Lower the bar slowly until it just touches your chest below the pectoral muscles. Keeping the elbows pointed outward, press the bar upward until your arms are locked out.

Variations

One-Arm Bench Press

You can't perform free-weight barbell bench presses with one arm—at least safely. Here's another situation where the Smith Machine shines, providing the tracked movement for some unilateral pressing. You may discover something by doing this.

Tips & Technique

- This is the king of ego lifts for men. Don't fall prey to the siren song of bigger weights until you can handle them in good form. This bench press is not immune to the benefits of progressive resistance and tends to reward those with patience and perseverance.

- As you widen your grip, the range of motion decreases, as does the direct involvement of the triceps. However, the stress on the shoulders increases. Keep this in mind if you are dealing with any shoulder issues.

- For some individuals, different upper arm angles will produce better or worse results, mostly based on your anthropometry—how you are built. Experiment with your arms outward at 45-degree angles from your body or in closer to determine which produces the best results for you.

Guillotine Press

Builds mass and strengthens the upper pectorals.

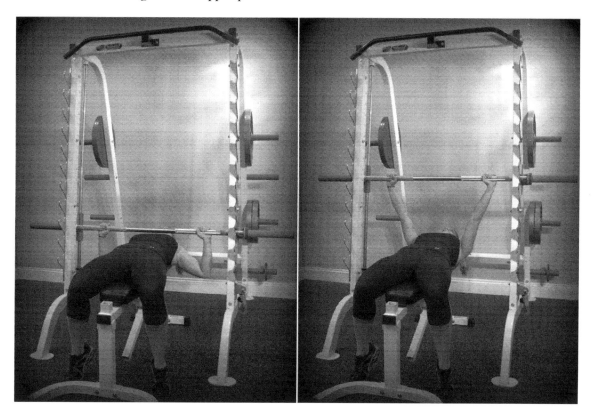

Performance

Place a flat bench under the Smith Machine bar. Set the safeties just above the height of the bench. Lie on the bench, grab the bar with a shoulder width (or wider) grip and unhook the bar. Slowly lower the bar until it's just above your collarbone. You should feel your upper chest stretch out. Keeping the elbows pointed outward, press the bar upward until your arms are locked out.

Variations

One-Arm Guillotine Press
Again, the rails-based system of the Smith Machine allows you to perform a unilateral version of this exercise effectively.

Tips & Technique

- Always set the safeties before starting this exercise, otherwise you may kill yourself. This is a highly dangerous exercise, unless proper safety precautions are always followed. You have been warned.

- Like the executioner, the Guillotine Press requires precision—otherwise, your shoulders are going to rebel against you. Your upper arms should remain perpendicular to your torso and in line with the bar on this exercise, as pictured above. This minimizes stress on the front of the shoulders and targets the upper chest.

- Try gripping the bar with your hands at a 45-degree angle to the bar (this forces the elbows out and the upper arms in alignment with the bar). This is a favorite movement of Larry Scott, the first Mr. Olympia bodybuilding winner, as described in his book, *Loaded Guns*. Larry had a genetically weak upper chest and this was one of the key exercises he used to enhance the development in that area.

Decline Press

Builds mass in the lower pectoral muscles.

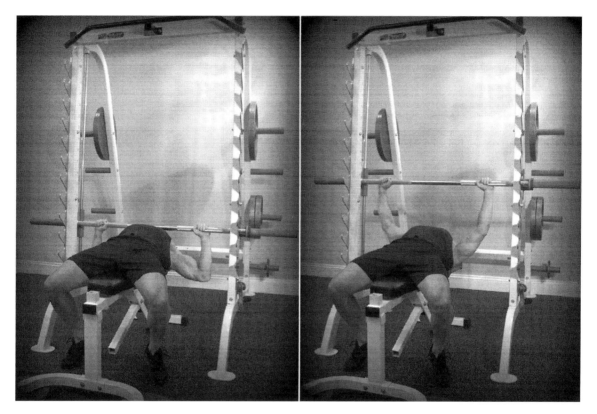

Performance

Place a decline bench under the Smith Machine bar. (If you don't have a decline bench, place a 45lb plate under the end of flat bench to create a slight decline.) Set the safeties just above the height of the bench. Lie on the bench with your head at the low end, grab the bar with a shoulder width (or slightly wider) grip and unhook the bar. Slowly lower the bar until it just touches your chest below the pectoral muscles. Keeping the elbows pointed outward, press the bar upward until your arms are locked out.

Variations

One-Arm Decline Press
The Smith Machine offers one of the rare venues where you can perform decline pressing with a single arm.

Tips & Technique

- The Decline Press is a useful exercise if you reach a plateau with the standard bench press. Due to the limited range of motion, compared to that exercise, most individuals will be able to press more weight here. This can help you both physically and psychologically in the short-term. Just don't get caught up in the clever trap of consistent decline pressing—your ego may get a short-term boost, but the long term effects on your body may not be what you want.

- If your bench can be set at a 45-degree decline, this will help you simulate a traditional dipping bar exercise for your chest.

- Try experimenting with closer and wider grips on this exercise. Closer grips will increase the range of motion, whereas wider grips will decrease it. Each of these grips becomes important depending on the current health of your shoulders (injured shoulders respond well to closer grips) and your immediate goal.

- For some individuals, different upper arm angles will produce better or worse results, mostly based on your anthropometry—how you are built. Experiment with your arms outward at 45-degree angles from your body or in closer to determine which produces the best results for you.

Floor Press

Builds strength in the chest.

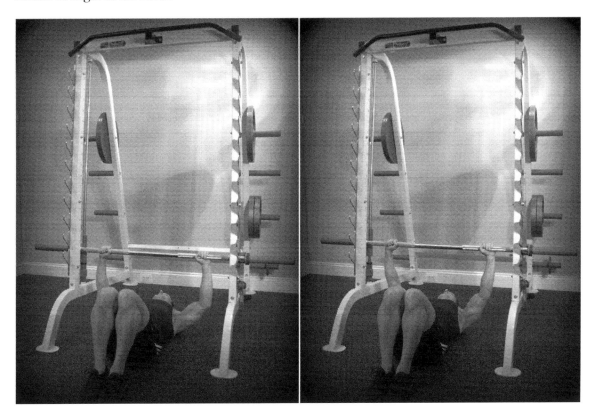

Performance

Lie on your back directly under the Smith Machine bar and grab the bar with a shoulder width (or slightly wider) grip. Unhook the weight and lower the bar until your triceps contact the floor. Pause and then press the weight back up. This exercise will help to develop maximum strength in the upper range of the bench press.

Variations

One-Arm Floor Press

We've talked enough here about the benefits of unilateral pressing, so you know by now it's a smart thing to do from both a balance and corrective perspective.

Tips & Technique

- This is an oft-forgotten movement, used in the era before standard exercise benches and dedicated bench press stations became common. It's also a favorite move of Bill Pearl, five-time Mr. Universe winner, as he describes in his seminal tome, *Keys to the Inner Universe*.

- Maintain control of the weight at all times here, especially as you lower it. You want your triceps to *lightly* contact the floor—not come crashing down and jarring joints.

- Although this exercise does limit the range of motion, it provides two benefits—learning to pause and hold the weight under tension and to drive the bar to lockout from that dead stop. Additionally, the partial movement here is beneficial for working through the sticking point of the standard bench press. So, what appears to some as a lazy or strange way to perform bench presses is actually a method to increase the generation of explosive pressing power. Here, power truly is in the eye of the beholder.

Incline Press

Develops the mass and strength of the upper chest and front deltoids.

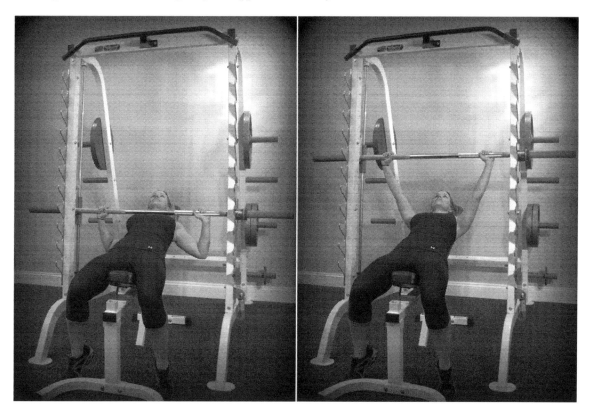

Performance

Place an incline bench under the Smith Machine bar. Set the safeties so that the bar will stop just below your chest. Lie on the bench, grab the bar with a shoulder width (or slightly wider) grip and unhook the bar. Lower the bar slowly until it just touches your upper chest. Keeping the elbows pointed outward, press the bar upward until your arms are locked out.

Variations

One-Arm Incline Press

Unilateral work is never a bad thing—and it can really help to teach you about feeling the muscles work—that all-important mind/muscle connection. Sometimes we tend to really concentrate with this type of work and—surprise, things start happening.

Close-Grip Incline Press

This variation provides two benefits—it helps those with bodybuilding and general physique aspirations fill in the difficult to develop region of the upper inner chest, and it provides a unique overload to the triceps muscles of the arms.

Tips & Technique

- There is much debate and disagreement over the most effective angle of incline to use—should it be 30, 40, or (gasp!) even 50 degrees? Here's the answer you've been waiting for—it depends. It depends on a lot of things, especially your anthropometry as defined by your structure, arm length, ribcage and shoulder width, etc. The key is to try each angle for a few weeks, note the results, and then move to a different angle and repeat the process. After a brief period of time (measured here in months), you'll have an individualized answer that can work optimally for you.

- A good tactic to employ if your incline press hits a plateau is to lower the angle of attack temporarily. This will allow you to handle a little more weight and increase the load. After a few weeks, revert back to your previous angle setting and you should be able to go right past that previous plateau. If not, see the **Intensity Techniques** section for more ideas.

Push-Ups

Develops the chest, triceps and shoulders.

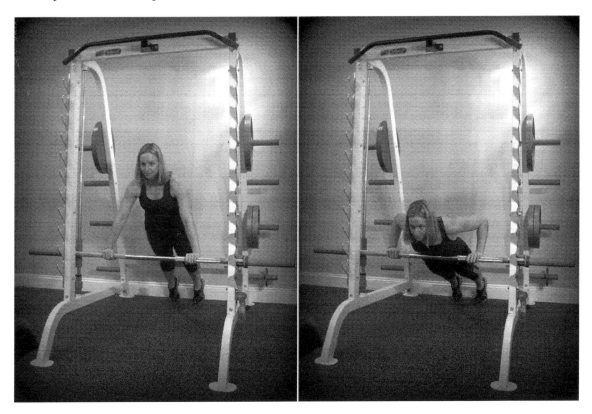

The push-up is one of the most basic exercises around. You probably learned how to do it in school gym class. Done consistently and correctly it works wonders, developing most of your upper body, including your chest, shoulders, arms and abs.

Performance

You can perform push-ups in a variety of ways, altering the intensity and range of motion. Here, you are going to use the height of the Smith Machine bar and your body position to alter the intensity and difficulty of the exercise. For the traditional push-up, place the bar of the Smith Machine at the lowest position. Grab the bar at shoulder width or slightly wider, keep your feet on the floor, torso straight and slowly lower until your chest touches the bar. Push yourself up until your arms are locked out. If you have trouble with this version, try supporting yourself on your knees instead of your feet. You can also raise the height of the bar slightly—this will reduce the difficulty of the exercise.

Variations

Close-Grip Push-Ups
By placing your hands closer than shoulder width, you increase the stress on your triceps as well as the inner chest.

Decline Push-Ups
Place your feet on an exercise bench instead of the floor. This increases the difficulty of the exercise. You can further increase the difficulty by wearing a weighted vest or backpack with this variation.

Kneeling Push-Ups
This is a useful variation if you are not strong enough to perform the exercise with your feet on the floor. Simply kneel down in front of the bar on your knees and perform the exercise as described above.

Tips & Technique

- It's essential to keep your upper and lower body straight throughout the movement. This helps work your abs as well, because you are essentially performing a moving plank. If you have trouble performing the exercise in this manner, you can perform push-ups with your knees on the floor or raise the height of the bar. Again, the higher the bar, the easier the resistance becomes.

-

Forearms

In general, you should attain good forearm development from holding onto progressively increasing weights with the Smith Machine bar when performing exercises such as deadlifts, rows and shrugs. However, if you weren't blessed with good forearm genetics, you don't use lifting straps on your exercises, and still have lackluster forearms, you'll need to incorporate some direct forearm work into your routine.

The key to maximizing forearm development is to treat them with as much emphasis as you place on your other muscle groups. Don't have time for this? Then, think about this—*any weight that you can wrist curl, you can bicep curl*. That should at least get the guys reading this motivated.

If you remember, the purpose of your forearms is to move your wrist up and down, so the exercises that you'll do for direct forearm work simulate those movements.

Here are the Smith Machine exercises to work your forearms:

- Wrist Curls
- Wrist Curls, Behind the Back
- Reverse Wrist Curls

A final tip: a great technique to bring up weak forearms indirectly is to perform a few sets of bar holds at the end of every workout. Set the safeties of the Smith Machine so that you can bend your knees slightly and lift the bar a couple inches when you stand back up. You just need to be able to lift the bar off the safety supports (one inch is fine). Load the bar with a weight that exceeds what you can do with shrugs, lift the bar and hold on until your grip gives out. Strive to increase the time or weight you can hold each workout. Repeat this a couple times a week and your forearms should catch up to the rest of your physique.

Wrist Curls

Develops the inside (flexor muscles) of the forearms.

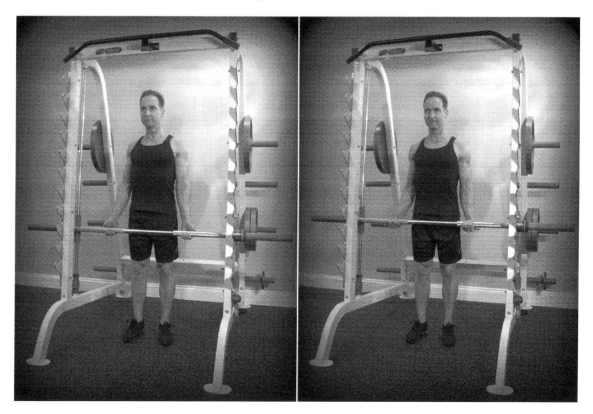

Performance

Set the bar of the Smith Machine just below arm's length, allowing your arms to hang straight down. Set the safeties just below that mark. Grip the bar about shoulder width or slightly wider. Let the bar roll down so that only your fingertips support the weight. Roll the weight back up into your palms and curl your wrists up as high as possible. Hold the contracted position for 1-2 seconds and slowly lower back down.

Variations

One-Arm Wrist Curls

If you are strong enough, you may want to try this unilateral version, which increases the intensity and is also a good variation for correcting a weaker forearm. Stand so your hand is positioned in the center of the bar (your body will be offset from the center of the machine).

Tips & Technique

- Because you use your forearms all day to pick up and hold things using a limited range of motion, the real key to forearm development is working through a complete range with progressive resistance.

- It's also important to keep your elbows and wrists on the same plane (whether sitting or standing) in order to maintain resistance throughout the movement. If standing, don't let your elbows move behind the vertical plane of your wrists—they should be straight above them. If sitting, make sure those elbows remain in contact with the bench at all times—this will ensure they remain on the same horizontal planes as the wrists.

Wrist Curls, Behind-the-Back

Develops the inside (flexor muscles) of the forearm.

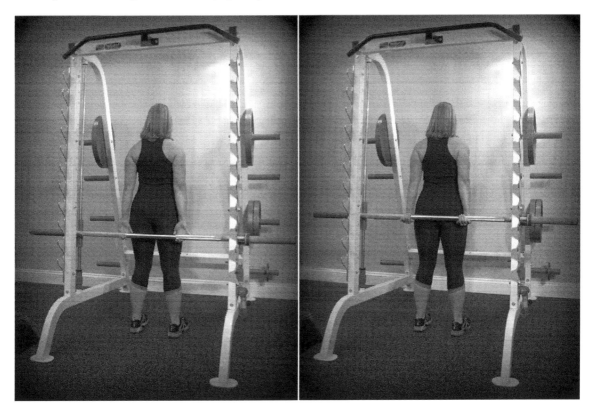

Performance

Set the bar of the Smith Machine just below arm's length, allowing your arms to hang straight down. Set the safeties just below that mark. Grip the bar behind your back, about shoulder width, with your palms facing to the rear. Let the bar roll down so that only your fingertips support the weight. Roll the weight back up into your palms and curl your wrists up as high as possible. Hold the contracted position for 1-2 seconds and slowly lower back down.

Variations

One-Arm Wrist Curls, Behind the Back

If you are strong enough, you may want to try this unilateral version, which increases the intensity and is also a good variation for correcting a weaker forearm. Stand so your hand is positioned in the center of the bar (your body will be offset from the center of the machine).

Tips & Technique

- This exercise becomes particularly effective when holding the weight on each rep in the contracted position for 2-3 seconds. Over time, using progressive resistance, your forearm flexors should become extremely strong and well developed.

Reverse Wrist Curls

Develops the outside (extensor muscles) of the forearms.

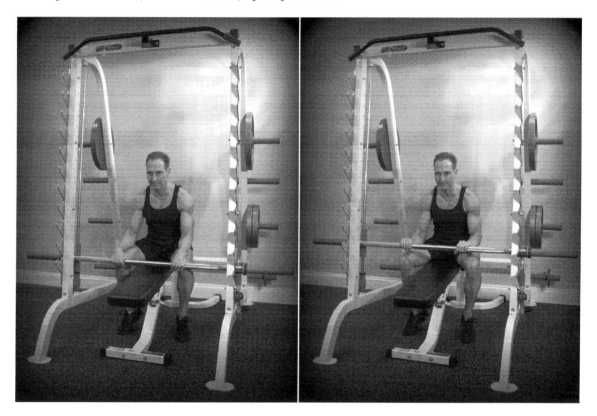

Performance

Place a bench under the Smith Machine and lower the bar onto the bench. Straddle the bench, and hold the bar with an overhand grip, hands close together. Sit down on the bench, resting your forearms on your thighs with your wrists hanging out over your knees. Bend your wrists forward as far as possible and then lift them up past parallel as far as possible. Hold the contracted position for 1-2 seconds, and then slowly lower.

Variations

One-Arm Reverse Wrist Curls
If you are extremely strong, you may want to try this unilateral version, which increases the intensity and is also a good variation for correcting a weaker forearm.

Tips & Technique

- This exercise becomes particularly effective when using a complete range of motion, because your forearms are not accustomed to full range extension with relatively heavy loads.

- Ensure that your elbows remain on your thighs throughout the exercise—don't allow them to rise up, because that will reduce the range of motion and remove much of the resistance. In times of stress, we always want to make the muscle work harder, and not give them the break they usually get in everyday activities.

- For some individuals, this exercise will be extremely difficult to perform correctly, given the combined weight of the empty bar and support mechanism. If you find yourself in this situation, either perform the one-arm variation using your free hand for assistance, or switch to Reverse Curls which can provide a similar effect.

Glutes

I like strong butts. If you're looking for the fabled fountain of youth, look no further. The glutes are it. Those glorious gluteus maximus muscles are the core of your body and the foundational power source for most of your movements. You need strong glutes. You want strong glutes. When you are 85, you'll thank me because you'll still be able to go to the bathroom on your own.

Typically, your glutes will develop in conjunction with your thighs, hamstrings and lower back when you perform squat, deadlift, and lunge movements. However, if you need extra work to increase glute size, power or shape, you can perform a special type of squat with a wide stance—the Duck Squat (sometimes referred to as the Frog Squat or a wide-stance squat).

Here are the important points for working your glutes effectively:

- Women (and men!) who squat deeply and consistently will develop glutes that can't be duplicated with other movements. Squats are the king (or queen!) of butt builders.

- When concentrating on this area, always squeeze your glutes as hard as possible at the midpoint of every glute-oriented motion—squats, lunges, and reverse lunges. Squeeze as hard as you think you can—then squeeze harder.

- Include both low rep sets with heavy weights and high-rep sets with lighter weights for maximum gluteal development. Glutes are both strong and durable so you've got to throw the entire repetition spectrum at them for full development.

With that out of the way, let's get to the Duck Squat.

Duck/Frog Squats

Works the glutes. Also works the thighs and hamstrings.

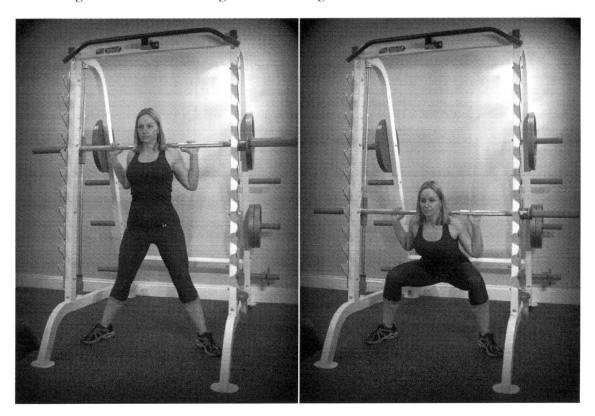

Performance

Lock the Smith Machine bar just below shoulder height and set the safeties at about mid-thigh. While standing, position the bar across your upper back. Place your feet several inches wider than shoulder width apart, pointing outward at 45-degree angles. Keeping your chest up and shoulders back, bend your knees and lower the weight until your thighs are just below parallel. Be sure to keep the center of gravity directly over your feet while not allowing the knees to go beyond your toes. Hold that position for a second, then push the weight back up, squeezing your glutes as you rise. At the top of the movement, squeeze the glutes hard again for a second or two.

Tips & Technique

- The same general tips apply to all forms of squats. Keep your chest up, back straight throughout, and your feet flat on the floor pointing slightly out. Make sure your knees travel directly over your feet and do not stray inward, especially as you ascend from the bottom of the movement. *Think knees out.*

- The real key to maximizing glute development is a full range of motion, proper form, and a hard squeeze of the glutes on each rep at the top for 1-2 seconds. Oh, and progressive resistance helps as well. Big weights build bigger, stronger butts. Ladies, don't be scared—I didn't say big, fat butts. Dietary control and cardio work is up to you.

Hamstrings

Hamstring workouts are built around concentric contraction-based exercises (some type of leg curl) and eccentric extension/hinge movements (some form of deadlift, such as Romanian or Stiff-Legged). The Smith Machine will allow you to perform both types of movements. Of course, your hamstrings are also heavily involved when you perform traditional squats (so keep doing them!).

For most people, hamstring development lags behind thigh development, sort of like the poor guy riding in the motorcycle sidecar. Not only does this make the legs appear incomplete and less shapely (hear that ladies?), but it presents a danger to athletes. Have you witnessed an athlete pulling a hamstring? It probably happened because the hamstring was asked to generate power that it didn't have.

Here are the important points for working your hamstrings effectively:

- Big, muscular hamstrings are built with a form of deadlift—not leg curls.

- If you have identified your hamstrings as a weak area, use the priority principle and work them at the start of your workout. Additionally, try working them *before* your thighs.

Here are the Smith Machine exercises to work your hamstrings:

- Romanian Deadlifts
- Stiff-Legged Deadlifts
- Straight-Leg Deadlifts
- Leg Curls

Romanian Deadlifts

Builds the mass of the hamstrings. Also works the lower back.

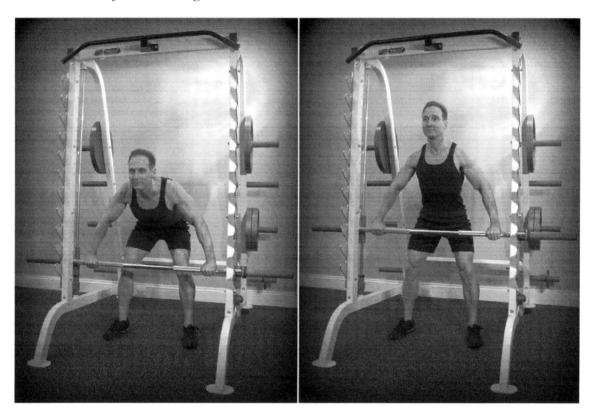

During the 1980s, Romanian Olympic powerlifter Nicu Vlad popularized the Romanian Deadlift, also called "RDLs". This unique form of deadlift places a large amount of stress on the hamstring muscles.

Performance

Set the safeties on the Smith Machine just below knee level so the bar rests there. Stand with your feet set at about shoulder width and grip the bar wider than shoulder width, using an overhand grip. Lift the bar by driving your hips forward and chest up, while keeping your shins vertical and your back straight. Lower the barbell to the starting position by pushing your hips back, keeping your chest up and back straight—you'll feel your hamstrings stretch in this position.

Tips & Technique

- Throughout the exercise, keep your back and arms straight and your shoulders pulled back.

- Unlike the Stiff-Legged or Straight-Leg Deadlifts, here your knees remain bent during the descent.

- A wider grip allows for a greater range of motion here. Not a bad thing.

Stiff-Legged Deadlifts

Develops the hamstrings, glutes and lower back.

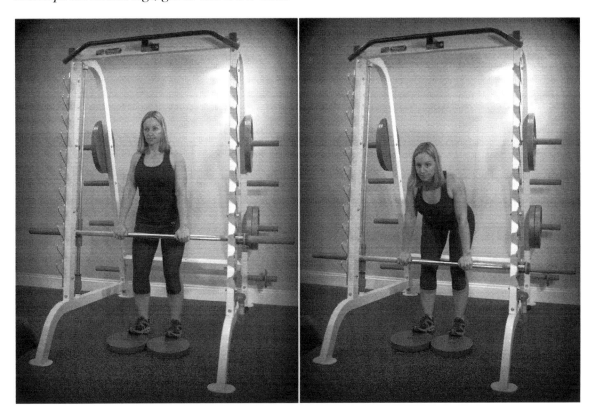

Performance

Set the Smith Machine bar at the lowest position (you won't need the safeties for this exercise). Bend forward at the waist keeping your back straight and your legs *slightly bent*. This will stretch your hamstrings. Grip the bar about shoulder width using an overhand grip. Lift the bar by extending the hips forward, keeping your back straight and the bend in your legs consistent throughout the movement. Slowly lower the bar to the starting position.

Variations

Close & Wide Stances

Because the hamstrings are a two-headed muscle, much like their upper body cousins the biceps, they respond well to changes in stance width, much like the grip widths on bicep curls. Wider stances place more stress on the inner muscle of the hamstring (semitendinosus), whereas narrower stances do the same for the outer long head (biceps femoris). Make sure to incorporate all stances (shoulder width, narrower and wider) into your overall hamstring program for complete development.

Tips & Technique

- Ensure your legs remain bent at a consistent angle throughout the exercise. A common mistake is to incorporate additional knee flexion (bending) while lowering the bar—that removes some of the stress from the hamstrings and helps defeat the purpose of the exercise.

- Throughout the exercise, keep your back and arms straight and your shoulders pulled back.

- Only lower the weight until your hamstrings are stretched—don't lower beyond a mild stretch. This range will differ from individual to individual, based on your current level of flexibility. Over time, you should be able to increase your range of motion.

- Stand on an aerobic step or two plates if the Smith Machine does not allow you to reach a full range of motion.

Straight-Leg Deadlifts

Develops the hamstrings, glutes and lower back.

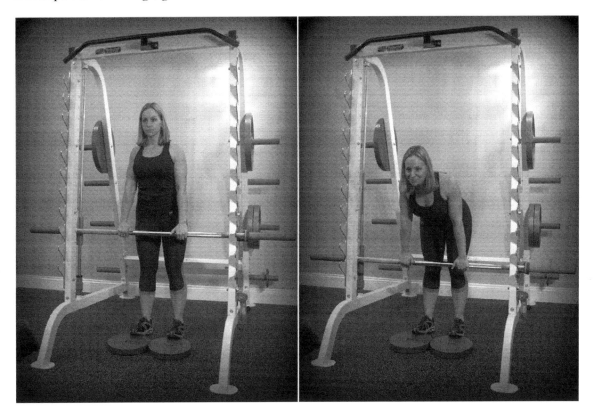

By keeping the legs straight in this exercise, more direct stress is placed on the hamstrings and lower back.

Performance

Set the safeties on the Smith Machine below knee level so the bar rests there. Stand with your feet set at about shoulder width and grab the bar with an overhand grip. Lift the bar to a standing position straightening the legs as you lift. Lock your legs straight and bend forward at the waist, keeping your back straight, until your hamstrings are stretched. Your arms should be holding the weight straight down in front of you. Return to the standing position, keeping your knees locked and the back straight.

Variations

Close & Wide Stances

Because the hamstrings are a two-headed muscle, much like their upper body cousins the biceps, they respond well to changes in stance width, much like the grip widths on bicep curls. Wider stances place more stress on the inner muscle of the hamstring (semitendinosus), whereas narrower stances do the same for the outer long head (biceps femoris). Make sure to incorporate all stances (shoulder width, narrower and wider) into your overall hamstring program for complete development.

Tips & Technique

- **Do not perform this exercise if you have any lower back issues**—the amount of direct stress placed on the spinal erectors of the lower back is significantly increased with the straight-leg version of this exercise.

- Throughout the exercise, keep your back and arms straight and your shoulders pulled back.

- Only lower the weight until your hamstrings are stretched—don't lower beyond a mild stretch. This range will differ from individual to individual, based on your current level of flexibility. Over time, you should be able to increase your range of motion.

- Stand on an aerobic step or two plates if the Smith Machine does not allow you to reach a full range of motion.

Leg Curls

Develops the leg biceps.

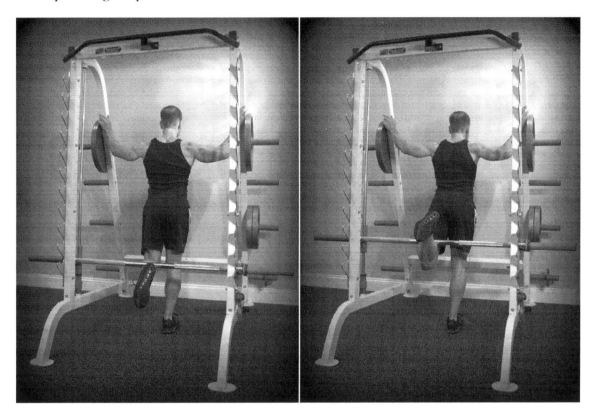

Performance

You will need either a thick towel or a barbell pad for this exercise. Set the safeties so the Smith Machine bar is set a couple inches below the back of your knees. Wrap the towel or barbell pad around the center of the bar. Place one of your legs under the padded bar so the bar is resting on your mid-calf. Curl your leg up by bending the knee as far as possible. Slowly return to the starting position and repeat. After you are finished, switch to the other leg and repeat the exercise.

Tips & Technique

- Position yourself so that the working leg is in the center of the bar (your body will be slightly offset from the center of the machine).

- Stand on an aerobic step or a barbell plate if the Smith Machine does not allow you to reach a full range of motion.

- Due to the mechanical limitations of the Smith Machine, this traditional arc-based movement will be reduced to a small subset (the middle range) of the full range of motion here, because the bar must travel in a linear path. Although this does provide some benefit, I encourage you to also incorporate any of the deadlift exercises in this section for more complete hamstring development.

- For some individuals this exercise will be extremely difficult to perform correctly, given the empty weight of the bar and support mechanism. If you find yourself in this situation, perform any of the deadlift exercises in this section as a substitute.

Quadriceps (Thighs)

There is just no way around this absolute truth—if you want exceptional legs, you must squat. The act of squatting is one of the most natural human movements. Half of the world's population squats for large portions of the day in order to plant or harvest crops. A properly executed, full squat is one of the best methods to strengthen the muscles and connective tissues around the knee. It also helps build the glutes, lower back, and hamstrings, making it one of the cornerstone exercises available.

Due to its original design and intent, the Smith Machine allows you to squat your heart out, with no spotter, and with no fear of failure. Strong, muscular and shapely legs are right there for your taking. But like most things in life, there is no free lunch—it will require some serious mental fortitude on your part because large muscle groups demand large efforts. Additionally, squatting on the Smith Machine provides a good alternative for those with mildly sore lower backs which welcome stabilization as a respite.

You can also perform various lunging movements on the Smith Machine, although those will do much less for your leg strength and development than the plethora of squat variations you can perform.

Here are some important points for working your thighs effectively:

- Because most modern Smith Machines present an angled bar path, slight foot positioning changes here can produce a myriad of stress alterations compared with free-weight barbell squats. You'll find you should place your feet slightly more forward of the bar than you would normally set up with free-weight squats (where you want the bar mid-foot). Find the right foot position first by using the empty, unloaded bar on the Smith Machine. Most beginners place their feet either too far back or forward of the bar.

- Unless you are intentionally performing Half Squats or Bench Squats, you need to squat down until your thighs are slightly below parallel. Regardless of what someone may have told you, a couple inches really do make a huge difference.

- Look at a point on the floor about 10-15 feet in front of you when squatting. Don't look up or straight ahead. Look slightly down. This really seems to help lock people into the movement.

- The knees need to remain out during the entire movement, because squatting is simply the act of the torso dropping straight down between your legs. As you push up and drive the floor away from you, keep forcing your knees to remain out. *Think knees out.*

- Try different foot stance widths when squatting. Feet shoulder width apart, wider than shoulder width, and narrower. You can alternate stances during the workout or from workout to workout.

- For the ultimate in squatting intensity, try high-reps squats (20 reps) or 21s—first seven reps the bottom half of the squat, next seven the top half, and the final seven the entire range of motion. Then, excuse yourself to the rest room. You won't get that feeling or similar results from a set of leg extensions.

Here are the Smith Machine exercises to work your quadriceps:

- Squats
- Squats, One-Leg
- Squats, Overhead
- Front Squats
- Bench Squats
- Bench Front Squats
- Split Squats
- Split Squats, One-Leg
- Hack Squats
- Jefferson Squats
- Zercher Squats
- Half Squats
- Sissy Squats
- Step Ups
- Lunges
- Reverse Lunges

Squats

Builds mass and strengthens the legs, especially the thighs.

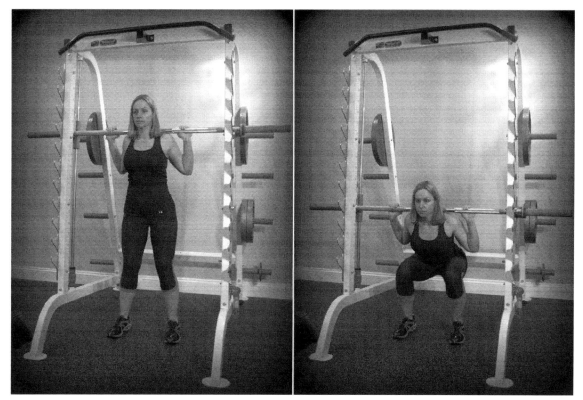

All hail the king of squatting movements! Master this, and you've mastered most of weight training, at least psychologically.

Performance

Set the safeties on the Smith Machine to just below waist level. Set the bar at shoulder height. While standing with a shoulder width stance, feet pointing slightly out, unhook the bar and position it across your upper back. Keeping your chest up, back straight and shoulders retracted bend your knees and move your hips back to lower the weight until your thighs are just below parallel. Be sure to keep the center of gravity directly over your feet while not allowing the knees to stray inward. Push the weight back up using your thighs.

Variations

Narrow and Wide Stances

A stance narrower than shoulder width will stress the outer thigh and stances wider than shoulder width stress the inner thigh. You are only as strong in the squat as your weakest stance so master them all.

Tips & Technique

- Like most good exercises, you really need to let your body dictate the natural movement. In essence, you squat between your legs. Keeping your chest up, just drop your torso straight down and allow yourself to sink between your legs. Don't overthink it.

- Keep your chest up, back straight and the weight squarely on the center of the feet. Varying from these positions invites injury.

- The feet can point straight ahead or outward at a 30 degree angle (preferred). Your knees should always follow the direction that your feet are pointing.

- Women who consistently squat as part of their weight training program develop legs and glutes that can't be duplicated with other movements, providing empowerment, strength and beauty in one exercise.

Squats, One-Leg

Builds mass and strengthens the legs, especially the thighs.

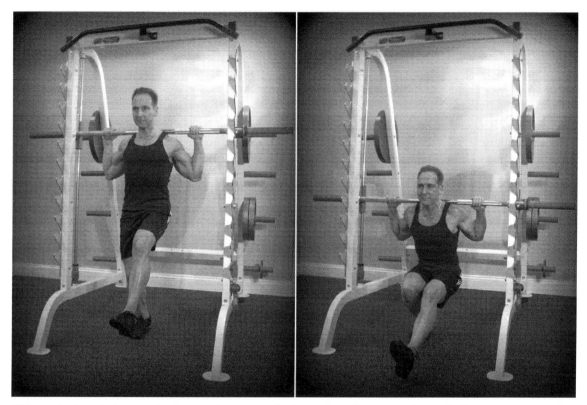

This variation of the standard squat increases the intensity of the exercise and allows you to check for and correct imbalances in strength and development of one leg versus the other. And it's damn hard to do.

Performance

Set the safeties on the Smith Machine to just below waist level. Set the bar at shoulder height. While standing with a shoulder width stance, unhook the bar and position it across your upper back. Shift your weight to one leg and lift the other leg out in front of you. Keeping your chest up, back straight and shoulders retracted extend your hips back and bend your knee to lower the weight until your thigh is below parallel. Be sure to keep the weight squarely on the mid-foot while not allowing your knee to go beyond your toes. Push the weight back up using your leg. After finishing your reps with one leg, repeat the exercise with the other.

Variations

One-Leg Bench Squats

Use this variation if the freestanding version is too difficult for you. Although this exercise may at first appear intimidating, the bench will initially provide you with the reassurance that you can perform the movement. Simply lower yourself slowly until your glutes contact the bench and then push back up.

Tips & Technique

- Keep your chest up, back straight, weight on the mid-foot and descend until the thigh is just below parallel. Make sure the knee tracks in the same direction the as the foot.

- Newcomers to this exercise may want to adjust the safeties so that you can start with a limited range of motion—say, halfway down and then proceed from there as you acclimate to the full range of the movement. Confidence and courage will propel you upward.

Squats, Overhead

Works the thighs, shoulders, triceps and abdominals.

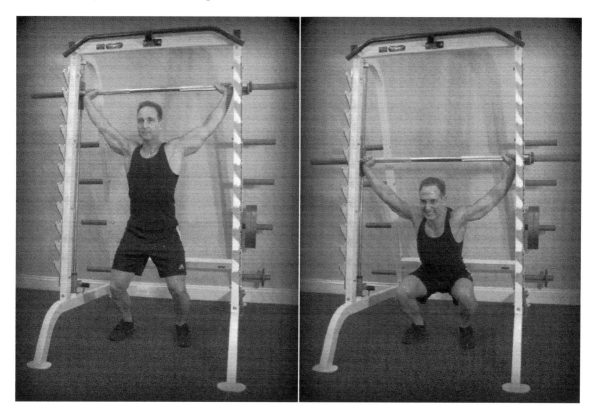

Performance

Lock the bar of the Smith Machine to the highest position you can reach. Stand under the bar, extend your arms and hold the bar at a position wider than shoulder width. Keeping your arms locked at the elbows, unlock the bar and squat down as deeply as you can as if performing a standard squat. Push the weight back up using your thighs. Keep the weight squarely on your mid-foot throughout this exercise.

Variations

Bench Squats, Overhead
For beginners, the bench can be used to help pattern the movement.

Tips & Technique

- Keeping the arms locked at the elbow and your traps shrugged will go a long way here. It also helps to use a wide stance for this exercise.

- Keep your chest up, back straight, and weight on the mid-foot. Make sure the knees track in the same direction the as the feet.

Front Squats

Works the legs with special emphasis on the thighs.

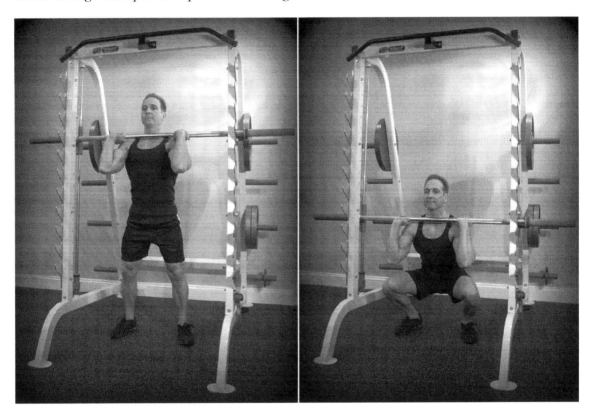

Although traditional squats work the quadriceps, hamstrings, lower back and glutes, the front squat squarely emphasizes quadriceps power, removing much of the involvement of the hamstrings and lower back. This can be useful for both the bodybuilder and those recovering from lower back issues.

Performance

Set the safeties on the Smith Machine to just below waist level. Set the bar at shoulder height. While standing with a shoulder width stance, feet pointing slightly out, unhook the bar and position it across your upper chest as if you are performing a shoulder press. Position the elbows as high as possible. Keeping your chest and elbows up and back straight, extend your hips back and bend your knees to lower the weight until your thighs are just below parallel. Push the weight back up using your thighs. Keep the weight squarely on the mid-foot throughout this exercise and the elbows up.

Variations

Narrow and Wide Stances

A stance narrower than shoulder width will stress the outer thigh and stances wider than shoulder width stress the inner thigh. For development of the outer thigh, nothing surpasses front squats with a narrow stance. You are only as strong in the squat as your weakest stance so master them all.

Tips & Technique

- In the photos above, the lifter is holding the bar using the traditional clean-style front squat grip. If you are not flexible enough to hold the bar in this position, use the bodybuilder's California-style grip with your arms crossed under the bar. Be aware, the California-style grip, although easier to use initially may limit the eventual amount of weight you can handle in this exercise, especially as you move to free-weight front squats. Try to work on increasing your flexibility using the traditional clean grip. Regardless of which grip you choose, the key here is to constantly force your elbows to stay up throughout the movement. This tends to keep everything else, like your chest, shoulders, hips and back, in proper position. *Think elbows up.*

- Keep your chest and elbows up, back straight, and weight on the mid-foot. Make sure the knees track in the same direction the as the feet.

- The feet can point straight ahead or outward at a 30 degree angle (preferred). Regardless, your knees should always follow the direction that your feet are pointing.

- Front squats are the movement that nobody wants to do (which is why you need to do them!) and are rarely seen in the gym, but boy do they make a difference. They're tough, as well as one of the harder athletic movements to master with weights. As such, they have direct carryover to athletic improvement.

- Think of it this way—traditional squats produce muscular thighs, glutes and hamstrings, whereas front squats give birth to muscular *and incredibly shapely thighs*. That's because this type of squat reduces the involvement of the glutes and hamstrings and puts it all on those thighs, allowing genetics to shine through. You can identify who performs this exercise consistently just by looking at their thighs.

- Due to the relatively vertical positioning of the torso on this exercise, front squats are much kinder to your lower back. Keep this in mind if you have any current low back issues.

Bench Squats

Builds power and size in the thighs.

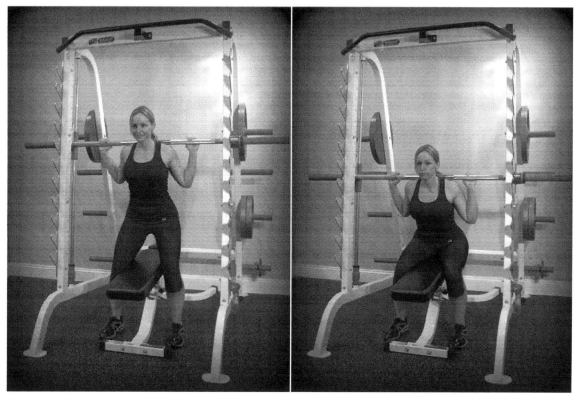

Bench Squats help you descend to a consistent depth when performing squats. They also increase your confidence to squat deeply as you progressively use shorter benches or boxes.

Performance

Place a bench directly under the bar of the Smith Machine. Set the safeties to just below waist level and the bar at shoulder height. While standing, straddle the bench, unhook the bar and position it across your upper back. Keeping your chest up and shoulders back, extend your hips and bend your knees to lower the weight until you gently sit on the bench. Stand back up by driving your hips forward while pushing with your thighs. Keep the weight squarely on the mid-foot throughout this exercise.

Tips & Technique

- Bench squats can be effective for increasing power at the bottom of the squat, teaching proper depth, and performing partial reps, depending on bench/box height. Optimally, you want three bench or box heights—one that places your thighs just below parallel, one at parallel, and another just above parallel. Working diligently at all three heights provides maximum benefit and carryover results to the standard squat.

- One warning about bench squats—the presence of the bench does not give you license to perform a free fall onto it. You want a controlled descent with a gentle sit at the bottom of the movement. Any sudden impact onto the bench can cause severe spinal compression from both ends—remember, you've got resistance on your back and at the bench, so be careful.

- Keep your chest up, back straight, and weight on the mid-foot. Make sure the knees track in the same direction the as the feet.

- The feet can point straight ahead or outward at a 30 degree angle (preferred). Regardless, your knees should always follow the direction that your feet are pointing.

Bench Front Squats

Builds power and size in the thighs.

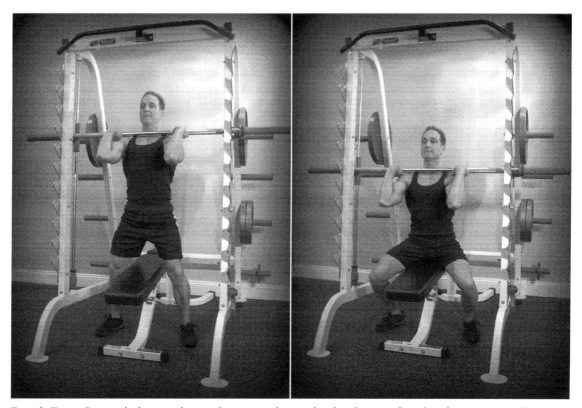

Bench Front Squats help you descend to a consistent depth when performing front squats. They also increase your confidence to squat deeply as you progressively use shorter benches or boxes.

Performance

Place a bench directly under the bar of the Smith Machine. Set the safeties to just below waist level and the bar at shoulder height. While standing with a shoulder width stance, feet pointing slightly out, unhook the bar and position it across your upper chest as if you are performing a shoulder press. Position the elbows as high as possible. Keeping your chest and elbows up and back straight, extend your hips back and bend your knees to lower the weight until you gently sit on the bench. Push the weight back up using your thighs. Keep the weight squarely on the mid-foot throughout this exercise.

Tips & Technique

- This exercise can be effective for increasing power at the bottom of the front squat, teaching proper depth, and performing partial reps, depending on bench/box height. Optimally, you want three bench or box heights—one that places your thighs just below parallel, one at parallel, and another just above parallel. Working diligently at all three heights provides maximum benefit and carryover results to the standard front squat.

- One warning about bench front squats—the presence of the bench does not give you license to perform a free fall onto it. You want a controlled descent with a gentle sit at the bottom of the movement. Any sudden impact onto the bench can cause severe spinal compression from both ends—remember, you've got resistance at both ends here, so be careful.

- Keep your chest and elbows up, back straight, and weight on the mid-foot. Make sure the knees track in the same direction the as the feet.

- The feet can point straight ahead or outward at a 30 degree angle (preferred). Regardless, your knees should always follow the direction that your feet are pointing.

Split Squats

Develops the thigh muscles. Also works the hip flexors.

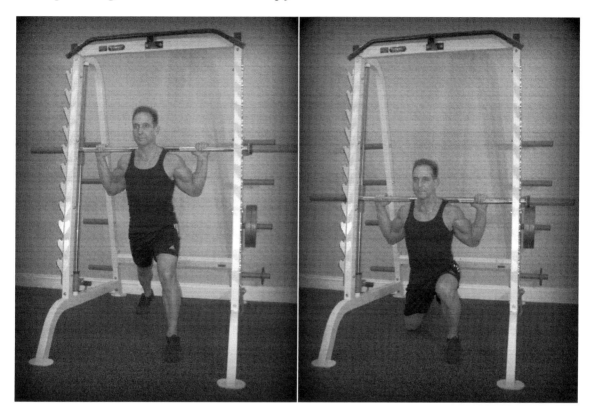

This movement is also known as Bulgarian Squats.

Performance

Set the safeties on the Smith Machine to just below waist level. Set the bar at shoulder height. While standing with a shoulder width stance, unhook the bar and position it across your upper back. Place one foot in front of the bar and the other back, until your rear heel is slightly off the floor. Slowly extend your hips, bend your knees and lower yourself until both legs are at 90-degree angles. Push the floor away from you using both legs until you reach the starting position.

Tips & Technique

- Keep your torso upright during the movement and your knee tracking in the same direction as your lead foot.

- The further your foot is in front of the bar, the more glute activation occurs. Conversely, the closer your front foot is to the bar, the more thigh involvement. Experiment with various placements of the front foot to attain your desired result.

Split Squats, One-Leg

Develops the thigh muscles. Also works the hip flexors.

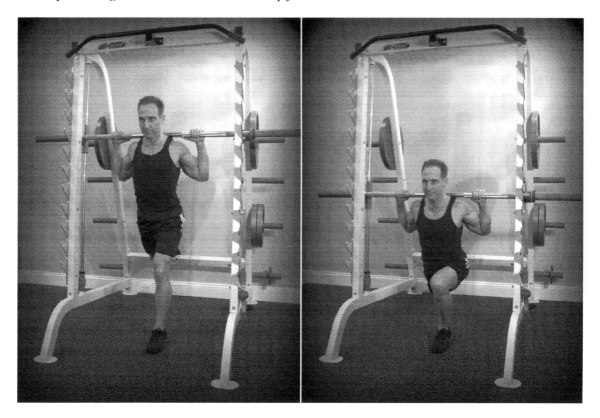

This movement is also known as Bulgarian Split Squats and is a more difficult version of standard Split Squats providing greater results.

Performance

Place a flat bench 2-3 feet behind the bar of the Smith Machine. Set the safeties on the Smith Machine to just below waist level. Set the bar at shoulder height. Unhook the bar and position it across your upper back. Place one foot in front of the bar and the top of your other foot on the bench. Slowly extend your hips, bend the knee and lower yourself until your lead leg is at a 90 degree angle or your rear knee is almost in contact with the floor. Using your lead leg, drive your hips forward and push the floor away from you until you reach the starting position. Continue for the prescribed number of reps, then switch legs and repeat.

Tips & Technique

▪ Some varieties of Smith Machine will have a horizontal stabilizing bar at the rear frame of the machine you can use to rest your rear foot on (as pictured above). If your machine doesn't include this feature, substitute an exercise bench or aerobic step for similar effect, as described above.

▪ Keep your torso upright during the movement and your knee tracking in the same direction as your lead foot.

▪ The further your foot is in front of the bar, the more glute activation occurs. Conversely, the closer your front foot is to the bar, the more thigh involvement. Experiment with various placements of the front foot to attain your desired result.

Hack Squats

Develops the thighs without putting too much stress on the glutes and lower back.

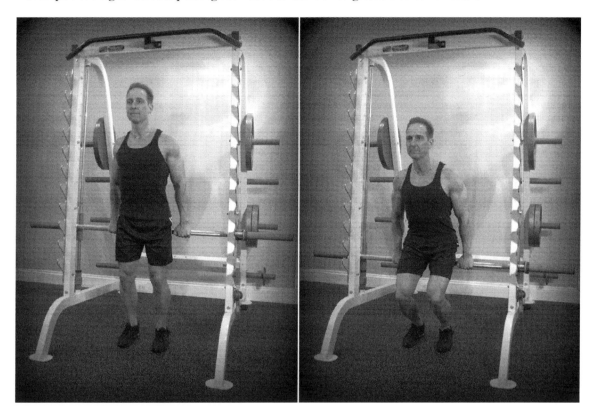

With the emergence of the dedicated Hack Squat machine, this exercise became relegated to the dust bin of weightlifting history. However, if you don't have access to a Hack Squat machine, this Smith Machine exercise can emulate its effect. It's also useful to take the stress off your lower back and place it squarely on your quadriceps.

Performance

Set the Smith Machine bar at arm's length when your arms are hanging straight down. You won't need the safeties for this exercise. While standing, hold the bar behind your back using an overhand grip. Keeping the bar pressed against your buttocks and your back straight, extend your hips and bend your knees to lower the bar as far as possible. Push the weight back up by driving your hips forward and extending the knees. Keep the weight squarely on the mid-foot rather than your toes throughout this exercise.

Variations

Narrow and Wide Stances

Vary your foot stance width from shoulder width to narrower and wider placements periodically. This will aid in the epic struggle to progress forward.

Tips & Technique

- You may need to stand on an aerobic step or two plates to achieve a greater range of motion here.

- Keep your hips low, arms and back straight and shoulders retracted during this exercise. Make sure the knees track in the same direction the as the feet.

- This is a great exercise to stress the outer thigh, much like the Front Squat. It works particularly well when combined with continuous tension—don't ascend all the way up on each rep, until your set is over.

Jefferson Squats

Develops the thighs and glutes without placing undue stress on the lower back.

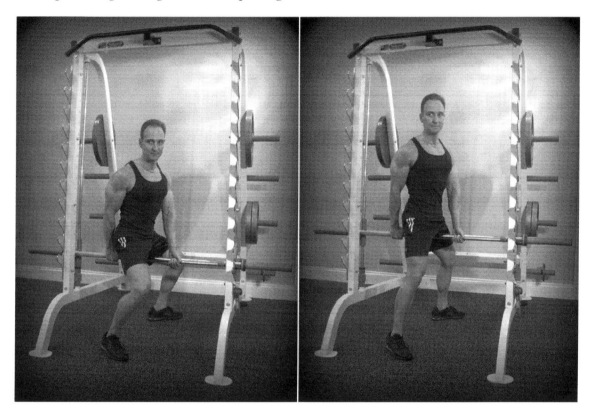

In the late 19th century, Barnum & Bailey circus strongman Charles Jefferson popularized this unique form of lifting a weight using a squatting movement. This is a largely forgotten, powerful move that will strengthen and develop your hips and legs. Here's how you do it today using the Smith Machine.

Performance

Set the bar of the Smith Machine at the lowest position. No need to hook the bar or use the safeties. While straddling the bar, bend your knees so that you grip the bar with one hand in front of you and the other behind. Now stand up while holding the bar making sure to keep your back straight and as erect as possible. Slowly lower to the starting position.

Variations

Goblet Squat

If you hold the bar with both hands in front of you, arms hanging straight down, you can morph this exercise into a goblet squat—one of the best exercises to teach the movement pattern of the full squat. Goblet squats are all kind of useful for understanding that squats are about lowering your torso between your legs and not folding/unfolding your knees.

Tips & Technique

- The Jefferson Squat is an excellent exercise to force your thighs to adapt by taking them to complete failure, while sparing your lower back from the drama. Because the weight is not supported by your back you can keep squatting until you can't stand back up. Couple this exercise with the Drop Set intensity technique and you've really got something that can demand adaptation to occur.

- Use this exercise if you are recovering from low back issues. Don't use it as a weekly staple— that's what squats and front squats are for.

Zercher Squats

Develops the thighs and glutes without placing undue stress on the lower back.

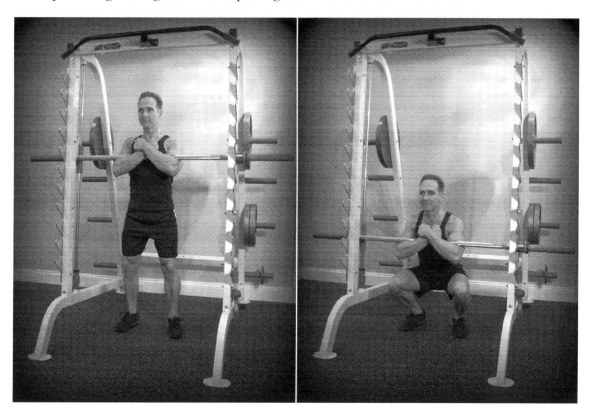

Strongman Ed Zercher popularized this unique form of squat in the early 20th century. It's also a good introduction and gauge of just how difficult it must be to lift the Husafell Stone, should you yearn to compete in strongman competitions. Here's how you do it today using the Smith Machine.

Performance

Set the safeties of the Smith Machine just above the level of your knees. Set the height of the Smith Machine bar at waist level. Position the bar in the crook of your arms. Your knuckles should face the ceiling and your elbows should be held close to your body. Slowly lower yourself until your elbows touch your thighs. Push the weight back up by driving your hips forward and extending your knees. Keep the weight squarely on the mid-foot throughout this exercise.

Tips & Technique

- Initially you may want to give up on this exercise. Having a weighted bar in the crook of your arms when lowering and raising yourself is not a pleasant introduction to anything. But stay at it. The movement pattern will become more natural, your body (and arms) will adapt and you'll have a new friend in the arsenal you can use whenever that nasty low back interloper intrudes.

Half Squats

Develops extra mass and power in the thighs.

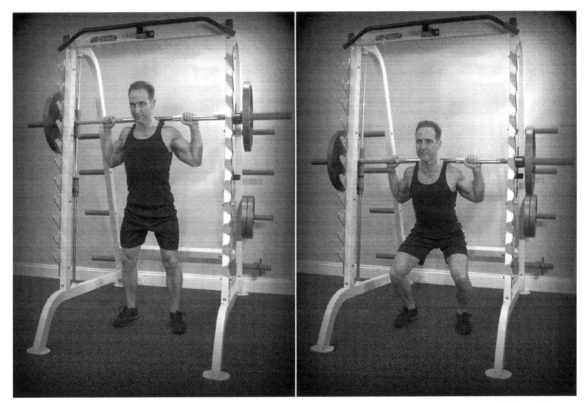

Half Squats are performed exactly like standard squats, except you use much more weight and descending only halfway, making sure to not lock out your knees at the top of the movement, in order to provide continuous tension on the thighs. This exercise builds hip power and upper leg mass.

Performance

Set the safeties on the Smith Machine to just below waist level. Set the bar at shoulder height. While standing with a shoulder width (or wider) stance, unhook the bar and position it across your upper back. Keeping your chest up and shoulders back, extend the hips and bend your knees to lower the weight until your thighs are at a 45-degree angle to the floor (halfway down compared to a standard squat). Push the weight back up using your thighs. Keep the weight squarely on the mid-foot throughout this exercise.

Variations

Narrow and Wide Stances

A stance narrower than shoulder width will stress the outer thigh and stances wider than shoulder width stress the inner thigh. You are only as strong in the squat as your weakest stance so master them all.

Tips & Technique

- Purposely using a partial range of motion on squats is useful for several reasons—first, it helps you psychologically handle some really heavy weights, typically weights you can't currently move through a full-range. Overcoming these types of mental hurdles is often the key to successful weight training. Second, it helps build explosive power in the hips (as do deadlifts) and add muscle mass to the upper portions of your thighs. However, exclusive use of half squats in your squatting repertoire is a common, classic mistake of beginners as well as advanced lifters with issues of ego, denial and hubris.

- Keep your chest up, back straight, shoulders retracted and the weight squarely on the center of the feet. Varying from these positions invites injury.

Sissy Squats

Isolates the lower quadriceps.

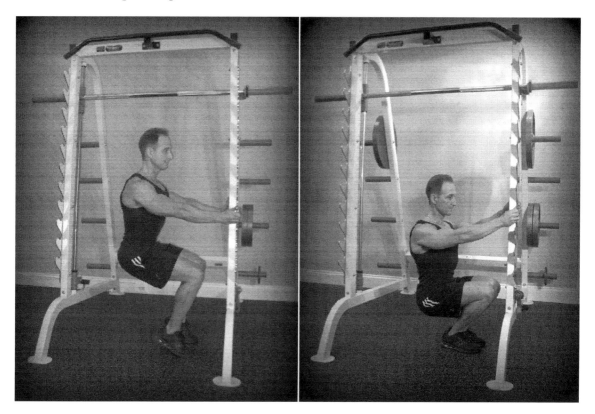

You can use the bar or frame of the Smith Machine to perform this body weight exercise.

Performance

While holding onto the bar (set at hip height) or machine frame for support, keeping your hips and waist straight, bend your knees and allow your body to lean backward as your knees move forward. Allow your heels to rise from the floor. Continue lowering your body (slowly) as far as possible without losing your balance. While maintaining this backward leaning position, slowly push back up using your thighs. Rise up only three-fourths of the way to the starting position and then repeat.

Tips & Technique

- You can increase the load and intensity by holding a small weight in one hand close to your chest or by wearing a weighted vest or backpack.

- Best results are achieved with a slow tempo and high reps (15+) on this exercise.

- Form is crucial for optimal results here—keep a straight back, lean backwards, and rise up on the toes while keeping constant tension on the thighs

Step-Ups

Develops the entire thigh and glutes.

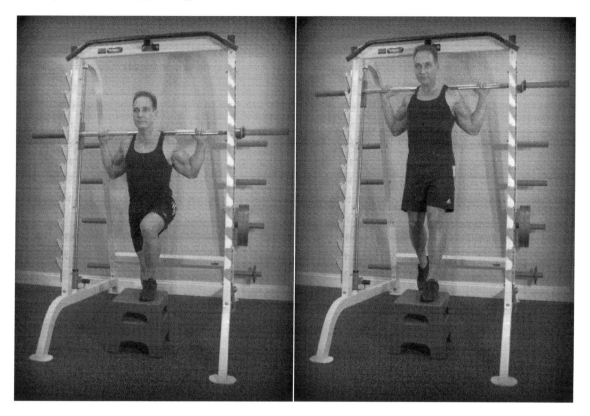

Performance

Place an exercise bench or aerobic step directly under the center of the Smith Machine's bar. Place your left foot on the bench and proceed to stand on the bench with both legs. Step down from the bench by lowering your right foot to the floor. Repeat for the desired number of reps, then lead with the other leg and repeat the process.

Variations

Alternating Step Ups

Instead of performing all of your reps with one leg then switching to the other leg, you can alternate legs each rep.

Tips & Technique

- Shorter benches or boxes make this exercise easier, whereas taller ones make it harder. Combine weight increases on the bar with the use of higher steps to achieve optimal progressive resistance here.

- The closer the bench or box is to the bar the more thigh involvement. Conversely, the farther away the bench or box, the more glute involvement occurs. Unfortunately, due to the constrained nature of the Smith Machine you are limited to how far away you can effectively place a bench or box.

- One common mistake is to lean forward when performing this exercise. Keep your chest up and back straight throughout.

- This exercise is a good alternative to Stiff-Legged Deadlifts for those with lower back issues.

Lunges

Develops the front of the thigh. Also works the hip flexors.

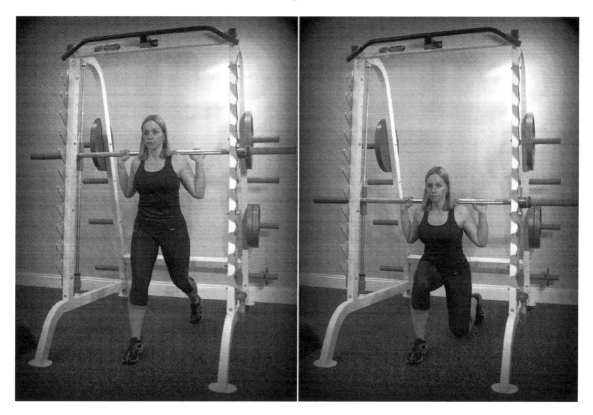

Performance

Set the safeties on the Smith Machine to about waist level. Set the bar at shoulder height. While standing, unhook the bar and position it across your upper back. Stand with your feet close together, keep your back straight and chest up, then take a step forward so that your leading leg is bent at a 90-degree angle to the floor, and lower yourself to the floor, landing first with your heel then forefoot. Be sure that the knee of the leading leg never goes beyond the toes. Push yourself back up to the starting position by extending your knee. After finishing your reps with one leg, repeat the exercise using the other.

Variations

Alternating Lunges
Instead of performing all of your reps with one leg then switching to the other leg, you can alternate legs each rep.

Tips & Technique

- Long lunges (taking a bigger step forward) emphasize the glutes and hamstrings, whereas shorter lunges emphasize the thighs.

- One common mistake is to lean forward while performing this exercise. Keep your chest up and back straight throughout.

Reverse Lunges

Develops the front of the thigh and the hamstrings.

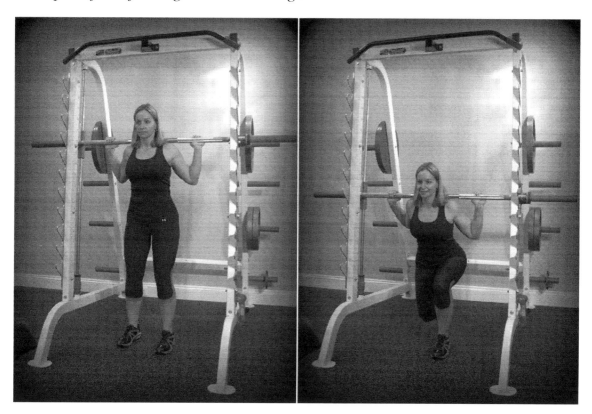

By stepping backwards in a lunge movement instead of forward, you increase the involvement of your hamstrings.

Performance

Set the safeties on the Smith Machine to about waist level. Set the bar at shoulder height. While standing, unhook the bar and position it across your upper back. Stand with your feet close together, keep your back straight and chest up, and then take a step back. Lower yourself until the knee of the rear leg is almost in contact with the floor. Push yourself back up to the starting position by moving your hips forward and extending your knee. After finishing your reps with one leg, repeat the exercise using the other.

Variations

Alternating Reverse Lunges

Instead of performing all of your reps with one leg then switching to the other leg, you can alternate legs each rep.

Tips & Technique

- Long lunges (taking a bigger step backward) emphasize more of the glutes and hamstrings, whereas shorter lunges emphasize the thighs.

- One common mistake is to lean forward when performing this exercise. Keep your chest up and back straight throughout.

Shoulders

Unlike your chest, back or calves, you can't escape from poorly developed shoulders, because they are visible from every angle and form the transaxle for all upper body exercises. Strong, healthy shoulders are also the key to performing most upper body activities in daily life, such as reaching, lifting and pushing things. I bet you use them a lot in your kitchen, bathroom and garage. Injure your shoulders or neglect them over time and your options become severely limited. Shoulders also represent the upper parapets of the classic Greek 'X' frame trifecta we've discussed. They are what makes that 'X' appear wide at the top and the intersection (your waist) seem so tiny in the middle.

Because the purpose of your shoulders (deltoids) is to lift your arms, they are developed primarily by pressing a weight overhead. You can also emphasize the front, side and rear muscles of your shoulders by performing various lateral raises to each of those sides. For optimum shoulder stability and health, you should work your shoulders from each of those angles equally in volume and intensity.

Here are the important points for working your shoulders effectively:

- Always try to start with a basic pressing movement to build overall strength and development of the entire shoulder complex before moving on to more isolation or indirect shoulder work.

- Use a full range of motion on shoulder presses. Don't stop lowering the weight at the top of your head. Build up your shoulder flexibility and lower the weight as far as you comfortably can. The importance of this will become more apparent as you age.

- Due to the over-emphasis in gyms on pressing movements in lieu of posterior chain pulling actions (again, mostly guys here—women seem to be much more adept as equal-opportunity lifters), the front head of the deltoid always seems to overpower the rear head. And imbalances like this are never a good thing for a sustainable weight training career. To correct these posterior deltoid imbalances, try performing rear delt rows after your presses. It may also be prudent to start your shoulder work with rear delt rows every couple of workouts. This will greatly assist the health of your shoulder's rotator cuff and labrum. If you don't know what those are, I'll just say you don't want to find out in your orthopedic surgeon's office.

Here are the Smith Machine exercises to work your shoulders:

- Military Press, Seated
- Military Press, Standing
- Push Press

- Press Behind the Neck
- Reverse Press
- One-Arm Press
- Front Raise
- Wide-Grip Upright Rows
- Heavy Upright Rows
- Bent-Over Rear Delt Rows

Military Press, Seated

Builds the overall shoulder structure with emphasis on the front deltoids.

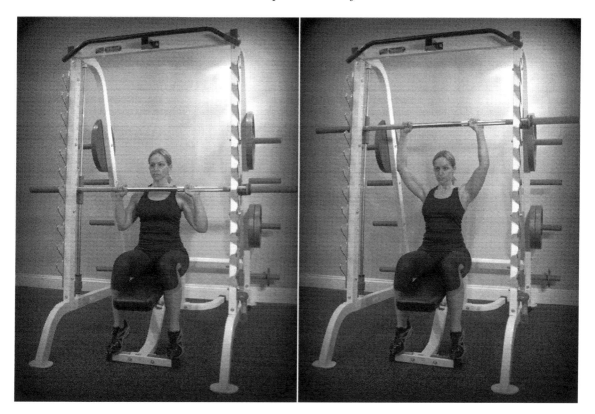

Performance

Place an exercise bench directly under the Smith Machine bar. While seated, set the safeties at just below shoulder height. Using a shoulder-width grip, unhook the bar and lower it to your upper chest. Press the bar overhead until your elbows are locked out. Slowly lower to the starting position.

Tips & Technique

- The seated version of the press is a useful alternative if you have lower back issues and cannot perform the standing version, because it provides more stability, but at the expense of core strengthening.

- Closer grips increase the range of motion, but also increase the amount of triceps involvement. Conversely, wider grips reduce range of motion and relative triceps involvement, but increase the stress on the connective tissues of the shoulder. Too wide of a grip here can be a bad thing. Aim for a grip width that results in your upper arms being perpendicular to the floor when the bar is at the starting position (see the picture on the left above). As always, experiment with an empty or lightly loaded bar to find your optimal grip width, based on your goals.

- It's also useful to experiment with using both a vertical torso and positioning an incline bench at a steep angle. Sitting back on a high-angled incline places more stress on both the front of the shoulders and the upper chest, an area which is often hard for many to fully develop.

Military Press, Standing

Builds the overall shoulder structure with emphasis on the front deltoids.

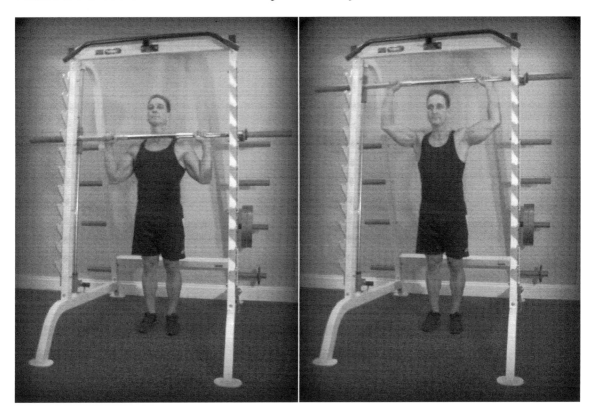

The standing version of the Military Press brings your core muscles (abs, obliques, lower back) into play. It's also one of the foundational exercises relished by both powerlifting and bodybuilding experts alike—a pure test of mind and might against gravity, fear and spirit with huge carryover effects to other pressing exercises. Pressing heavy weights overhead represents one of the true summits of weightlifting and helped both Atlas and the builders of the Farnese Hercules. It can do the same for you.

Performance

While standing, set the safeties at just below shoulder height. Using a shoulder width stance and grip-width, unhook the bar and lower it to your upper chest. Press the bar overhead until your elbows are locked out. Don't use your legs to assist with the press. Slowly lower to the starting position.

Variations

One-Arm Standing Military Press
This is a great variation to use when assessing symmetrical strength and development and performing corrective action. It also increases core activation, so you might notice some abdominal soreness the next day. That's a good indicator of the overall systemic effectiveness of this version.

Tips & Technique

- I realize most of us are lazy, but standing is where it's at. One of the tenets I always like to preach is "*sit if you must, otherwise stand if you can*". Try to incorporate that into your decision-making process with all exercise selections.

- You can stand with either the feet at shoulder width apart, or with one forward of the other. Try each type of stance and see which provides you with the most stability. As the weights increase on this exercise you may find the offset stance provides a more stable base and mirrors the Olympic lifter's stance when executing the final portion of the clean and press.

- If you are tall or your Smith Machine is short (many home versions are shorter than their commercial counterparts), the bar may reach the top of the rail system before you reach full extension. In these cases, you'll need to substitute the seated version of the exercise.

- Closer grips increase the range of motion, but also increase the amount of triceps involvement. Conversely, wider grips reduce range of motion and relative triceps involvement, but increase the stress on the connective tissues of the shoulder. Too wide of a grip here can be a bad thing. Aim for a grip width that results in your upper arms being perpendicular to the floor when the bar is at the starting position (see the picture on the left above). As always, experiment with an empty or lightly loaded bar to find your optimal grip width, based on your goals.

- This exercise forms the natural gateway to the Push Press, so master this movement before embarking on that route.

Push Press

Develops additional shoulder size and strength.

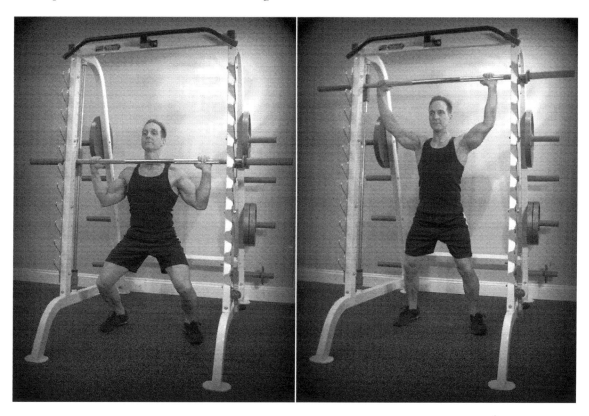

This version of the overhead press allows you to use a heavier than normal weight, or to continue to do repetitions of shoulder presses after reaching a point of failure with the strict Military variety. It also brings your core muscles (abs, obliques, lower back) and legs into play.

Performance

While standing, set the safeties at about chest height. Using a shoulder width stance and grip-width, unhook the bar and lower it to your upper chest. Dip your body slightly by bending your knees and then drive the bar overhead explosively, using your legs and arms in unison, until your elbows are locked out. Slowly lower to the starting position.

Tips & Technique

- This is a highly effective exercise to use immediately after you reach muscular failure with the strict standing Military Press. The Push Press allows you to push past those limits and recruit additional muscle fibers, resulting in more strength and development in the upper body. Alternatively, you can start with this exercise in order to overload your shoulders with a weight greater than you can use with strict standing Military Presses.

- You can stand with either the feet at shoulder width apart, or with one foot forward of the other. Try each type of stance and see which provides you with the most stability. As the weights increase on this exercise you may find the offset stance provides a more stable base and mirrors the Olympic lifter's stance when executing the final portion of the clean and press.

- If you are tall or your Smith Machine is short (many home versions are shorter than their commercial counterparts), the bar may reach the top of the rail system before you reach full extension. In these cases, you can stop just short of the top of the machine—you'll still get the benefit of developing starting explosive pressing power using the shoulders, triceps and legs.

- Closer grips increase the range of motion, but also increase the amount of triceps involvement. Conversely, wider grips reduce range of motion and relative triceps involvement, but increase the stress on the connective tissues of the shoulder. Too wide of a grip here can be a bad thing. Aim for a grip width that results in your upper arms being perpendicular to the floor when the bar is at the starting position (see the picture on the left above). As always, experiment with an empty or lightly loaded bar to find your optimal grip width, based on your goals.

Press Behind the Neck

Builds the front and sides of the shoulders.

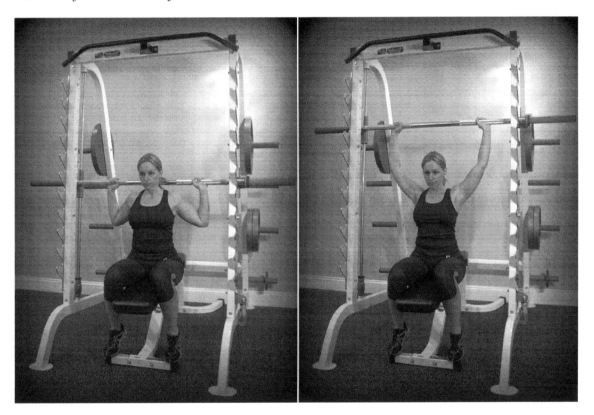

Performance

Place an exercise bench directly under the Smith Machine bar. While seated, set the safeties at shoulder height. Grip the bar slightly outside shoulder width, unhook the bar and lower it behind your head until the bar is at ear level or just below. Press the bar overhead until your elbows are locked out. Slowly lower to the starting position.

Variations

Standing Press Behind the Neck
By performing this exercise standing, the core muscles are activated. Just don't employ any push pressing tactics here—this exercise demands exacting form and control at all times.

One-Arm Press Behind the Neck
By switching to single-arm pressing, you can easily identify, assess and correct any imbalances in

strength and development in your overall shoulder structure. The intensity is also increased over the standard bilateral version.

Tips & Technique

- All weight training activities carry an inherent level of danger (as do *any* athletic endeavors). However, this is one of the more dangerous exercises you can perform, because it places the shoulder joint in a compromised position. As the weight is lowered, your shoulders move into extreme internal rotation—increasing the risk to the joint and your upper spine. There is little room for error here as you walk the razor's edge. However, performed with exacting form under complete control, this is an effective exercise for working the entire shoulder structure. I recommend using lighter weights, higher reps and a slower cadence on this one. If you don't have the shoulder flexibility or don't want to risk it, substitute the Seated Military Press instead.

- Closer grips increase the range of motion, but also increase the amount of triceps involvement. Conversely, wider grips reduce range of motion and relative triceps involvement, but increase the stress on the connective tissues of the shoulder. Too wide of a grip here can be a bad thing. Aim for a grip width that results in your upper arms being perpendicular to the floor when the bar is at the starting position (see the picture on the left above). As always, experiment with an empty or lightly loaded bar to find your optimal grip width, based on your goals.

Reverse Press

Builds mass at the front of the shoulders.

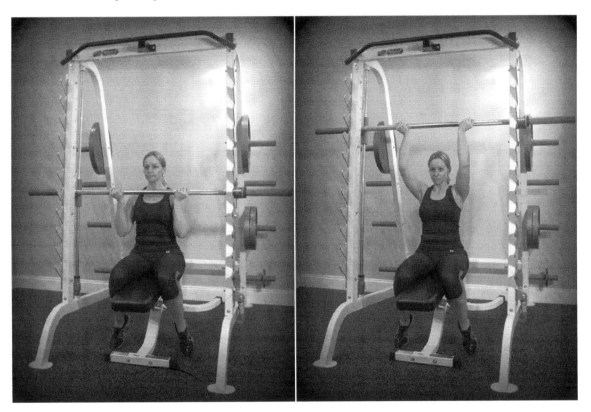

Performance

Place an exercise bench directly under the Smith Machine bar. While seated, set the safeties at just below shoulder height. Grip the bar at shoulder width with your palms facing you, unhook the bar and lower it to your upper chest. Press the bar overhead until your elbows are locked out. Slowly lower to the starting position.

Variations

Standing Reverse Press

By performing this exercise standing, the core muscles are activated. Again, taller lifters or those with shorter Smith Machines won't be able to achieve a full range of motion here.

Tips & Technique

- This is a largely forgotten exercise, popular with British bodybuilders in the 1970s and 1980s. It's also a good change of pace from Seated Military Presses, working some different assistive muscles in the process. You won't be able to use as much weight here as standard Military Presses.

- The first half of this movement largely mimics the classic Arnold Press using dumbbells. As such, the range of motion in this pressing movement is greater than with standard grip presses.

- Closer grips increase the range of motion, but also increase the amount of triceps involvement. Conversely, wider grips reduce range of motion and relative triceps involvement, but increase the stress on the connective tissues of the shoulder. Too wide of a grip here can be a bad thing. Aim for a grip width that results in your upper arms being perpendicular to the floor when the bar is at the starting position (see the picture on the left above). As always, experiment with an empty or lightly loaded bar to find your optimal grip width, based on your goals.

One-Arm Press

Develops mass in the shoulders.

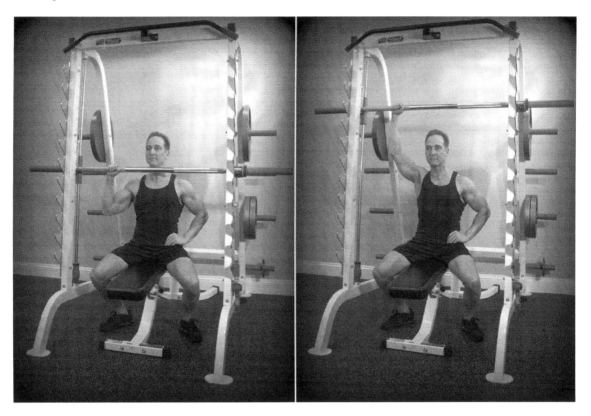

Performance

Place an exercise bench directly under the Smith Machine bar. While seated, set the safeties at just below shoulder height. Grip the bar at shoulder width using only one hand, unhook the bar and lower it to your upper chest. Press the bar overhead until your elbow is locked out. Slowly lower to the starting position. After completing the set, repeat with the other arm.

Tips & Technique

- This is a higher intensity version of the regular Seated Military Press, because all effort is concentrated on a single arm and deltoid. It also allows you to perform assisted reps with your free hand once you start reaching muscular failure with the working arm.

- Closer grips increase the range of motion, but also increase the amount of triceps involvement. Conversely, wider grips reduce range of motion and relative triceps involvement, but increase the stress on the connective tissues of the shoulder. Too wide of a grip here can be a bad thing. Aim for a grip width that results in your upper arm being perpendicular to the floor when the bar is at the starting position (see the picture on the left above). As always, experiment with an empty or lightly loaded bar to find your optimal grip width, based on your goals.

- It's also useful to experiment with using both a vertical torso and positioning an incline bench at a steep angle. Sitting back on a high-angled incline places more stress on both the front of the shoulders and the upper chest, an area which is often hard for many to fully develop.

Front Raise

Develops the front of the shoulders.

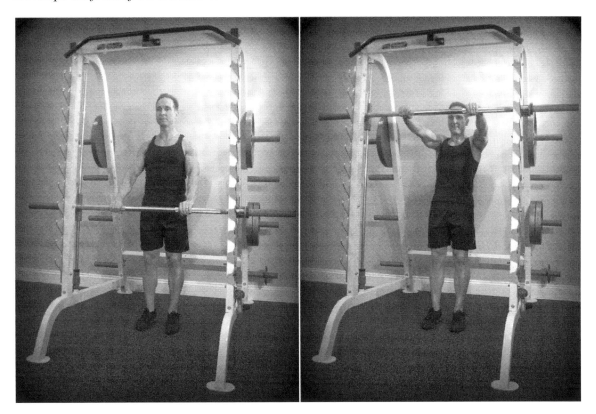

Performance

Set the Smith Machine bar at chest level and the safeties at waist height. Hold the bar at shoulder width with an overhand grip, keeping your arms straight and outstretched, so that you are a foot or two behind the bar. Unhook the bar and lift it until the bar is parallel to the floor, keeping your arms straight throughout. Slowly lower the weight and repeat.

Variations

Seated Front Raises

Performing front raises while seated is, of course, the strictest method possible, but at the expense of a more limited range of motion, due to bar contact with the thighs. This exercise will be challenging, even with an unloaded bar.

Reverse-Grip Front Raises

Using an underhand (reverse) grip works the area where the front of your shoulders and biceps connect. However, be careful to keep your arms relatively straight and use lighter weights or an unloaded bar. This variation, a past favorite of European bodybuilders, can strain biceps tendons if you're not careful.

Tips & Technique

- This is a difficult exercise to perform, even with an unloaded bar. If you can't do it, don't fret—lots of heavy pressing movements will build the front of your shoulders. If you are able to perform this move, try experimenting with different grip widths (from hands touching to grips wider than shoulder width) to discover which one works best for you.

- A close grip will activate some upper inner chest muscle fibers—not a bad thing, especially if you have a weakness there.

- The real key here is to keep your arms straight. Keep 'em straight and everything else will fall into place.

- You can also raise the bar higher than the parallel position. This will further activate the trapezius muscles, which is why you may feel some muscle soreness in the upper back the day after performing this exercise.

Wide-Grip Upright Rows

Builds the sides of the shoulders.

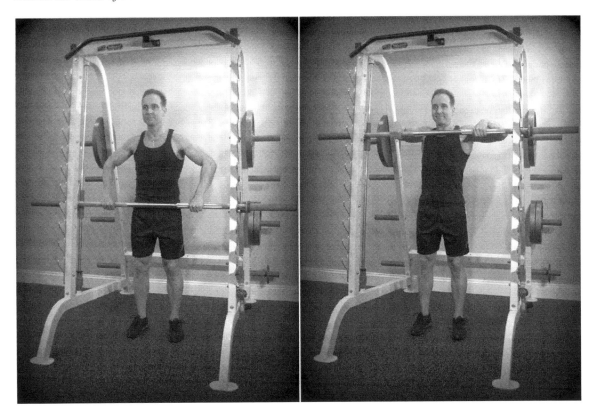

This exercise represents the best emulation of the traditional free-weight side lateral movement that you can perform on a linear-tracked Smith Machine.

Performance

While standing, hold the Smith Machine bar slightly wider than shoulder width, using an overhand grip. Pull the bar up until your upper arms are parallel with the floor. Slowly lower to the starting position.

Tips & Technique

- If you don't have access to dumbbells or cables, this exercise will allow you to emulate the lateral raising movement those objects allow.

- Grip width is critical here—grips either too wide or too narrow will reduce the effectiveness of the exercise. You want your upper arms on the same plane as the bar at the apex of the movement (see the picture on the right above).

- Concentrate on leading the movement with your elbows, keeping them slightly higher than your hands. *Think elbows high.* Make sure to squeeze and hold at the top position for a second before starting the controlled descent. Try to find the best grip width for your body structure—start with a high-rep set and notice how much fatigue you can induce in the side of your shoulders. That's what you're looking for.

- Don't raise your elbows higher than your shoulders—this can cause shoulder impingement injuries.

Heavy Upright Rows

Strengthens the entire shoulder girdle and upper back.

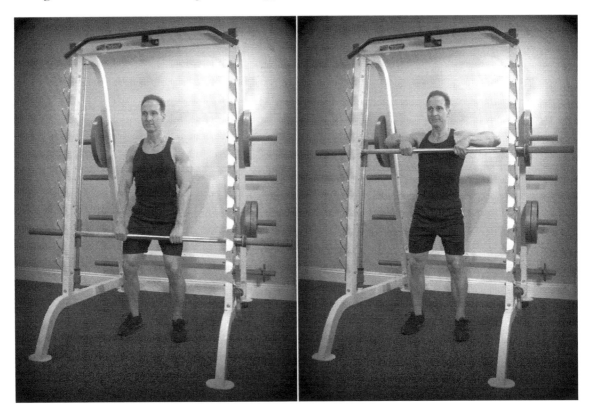

This is a heavier, cheating version of the standard Upright Row, allowing you to overload the entire shoulder structure, trapezius and upper back.

Performance

While standing, hold the Smith Machine bar with an overhand grip at about shoulder width. Pull the bar up, keeping it close to your body, until the bar is reaches upper chest height (good) or is just below your chin (great). You can cheat by using your legs on this exercise. Slowly lower to the starting position.

Tips & Technique

- These are not High Pulls—the key difference is that your grip will be closer here, the pull should be at a constant, almost rhythmic tempo and there should be minimal leg and hip drive.

You want to pull the weight up using upper body strength, with a little assistance from the legs as necessary.

- This is a useful exercise when you reach a plateau with standard upright rows or wide-grip upright rows, because the additional leg assistance and looser form allow for slightly heavier weights to be used. The carryover effect to those exercises should be noticeable.

Bent-Over Rear Delt Rows

Develops the rear of the shoulders.

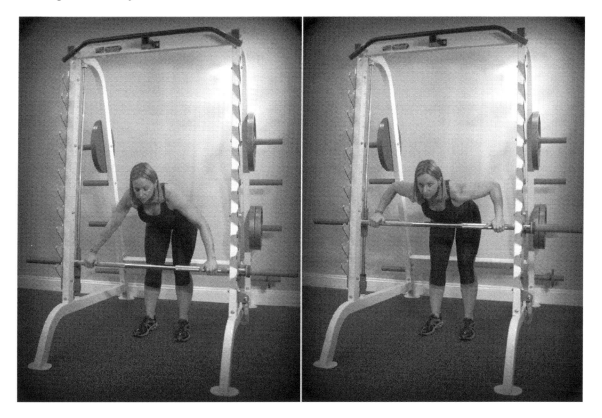

This exercise represents the best emulation of the traditional free-weight rear lateral raise movement that you can perform on a linear-tracked Smith Machine.

Performance

Set the Smith Machine bar at the lowest position. Bend over at the waist until your upper body is parallel with the floor. Hold the bar with an overhand grip slightly wider than shoulder width. Keeping your elbows in line with the bar, pull the bar up until it is near your chest. Squeeze your upper back, and then slowly lower to the starting position.

Variations

Supported Low Incline Rear Delt Rows
Use an incline bench set at a low (10-20 degree) angle so the bar is below the upper portion of the

bench pad. Lay face down and pull upwards using the instructions above. This is a great alternative if you are experiencing low back issues.

Tips & Technique

- You won't be able to use much weight (if any) on this one. That's not the point. The rear deltoid is a relatively small muscle and can be overloaded with little weight if perfect form, a high pull, and full contraction are used. Exacting form will produce the greatest results here.

- The key points are to keep your elbows and upper arms in line with the bar, use a slow, controlled pull ending with a paused contraction. You'll know you've accomplished this if you feel a pump in the rear of your shoulders and across your upper back.

Trapezius

Because your trapezius, ("traps") lift your shoulders up, they are important muscles for both men and women. By now, it should be no surprise they are developed with pulling movements, primarily various forms of shrugs and upright rows, although any type of deadlift or row will develop this muscle group over time. Ladies, this is not an area to neglect. Remember, the body is a unit and any part left untouched and undeveloped tends to cause other areas to become imbalanced. In this case, your traps comprise a large portion of your upper back and act as antagonists to your chest muscles. Pulling motions help to stretch the chest, and specifically, shrugging motions help to strengthen the neck and shoulders as well.

Here are the important points for working your traps effectively:

- The bulk of direct trap workouts should be with weights that you can perform through a full range of motion. Trapezius muscles respond well to extreme motion; therefore, you'll need to get those traps shrugged as high as you can and hold them in that position for a second or two.

- For those wanting or needing more muscle mass on the traps, then heavy weight is the way to go. Try using supramaximal weights that are so heavy you can't perform a full range of motion—but only use this type of training periodically.

- Concentrate on keeping your arms straight when shrugging—otherwise, you are sacrificing some trap activation and bringing the biceps into play. The arms don't need to be locked, just be cognizant of your form when doing these. If you notice your arms bending excessively, check the width of your grip on the bar—too narrow of a grip invites bent arms and the specter of bicep injury.

- Don't rotate your shoulders backward at the top of the shrug—that's not the function of the trapezius and can cause injury to the rotator cuff and labrum when using heavy weight. Your traps respond best to pulls on a linear plane, whether vertical, horizontal or at an angle in between. That's what makes the Smith Machine so ideal for shrug-based exercises.

- Try not to use lifting straps when performing shrugs or upright rows. When you get to the point where your grip is causing you to fail AND you are using extremely heavy weights, then it's ok to strap up.

- Avoid the three common mistakes of shrugs—bending your arms, using a limited range of motion (too much weight), and rotating your shoulders back at the top of the movement.

- Typically, you shouldn't need to perform any targeted exercises for your neck. If you are performing heavy deadlifts and shrugs on a consistent basis, your neck size should increase accordingly.

- For those seeking increased intensity for shrugging exercises, Drop Sets make the perfect lovers—often they spark instant chemistry and work well in the short-term. This technique allows you to use a heavy weight for 4-6 reps to increase muscular power and size in the traps, immediately followed by a lighter weight for 10-15 reps for muscular endurance. Because traps respond well to these extreme weight/rep ranges, drop sets give you the best of both worlds in a single set.

- Another effective technique for increasing intensity and finishing off your direct trap work is to shrug the bar up to full contraction and just hold it in that position, watching the clock. (This technique is called Static Holds.) Continue holding until your grip or your traps completely fatigue. Try to increase your hold time by at least one second each time you do this with a particular weight.

- Free weight devotees rehabilitating sore lower backs will find shrugs on the Smith Machine a useful respite for general stability, especially the seated and supported shrugs versions.

Here are the Smith Machine exercises to work your traps:

- Shrugs
- Shrugs, One-Arm
- Shrugs, Behind the Back
- Supported Shrugs
- Seated Shrugs
- Upright Rows
- Upright Rows, Behind the Back
- High Pulls

Shrugs

Develops the trapezius muscles.

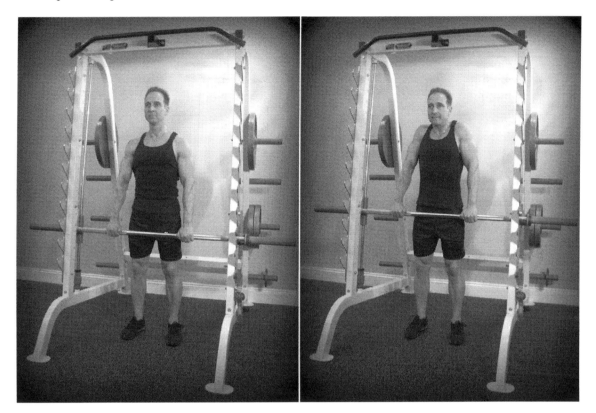

Performance

While standing, hold the Smith Machine bar in front of you with an overhand grip set at shoulder width or slightly wider. Keep your arms straight and raise your shoulders as high as possible. Hold for a second and slowly lower to the starting position.

Tips & Technique

- Experiment with different grip widths—in general, a narrow grip facilitates arm bending when pulling—something you may not necessarily want if you're trying to isolate the stress onto your traps.

- Don't forget the key points of shrugging—keep your arms straight, use a full range of motion, hold the contraction at the top for a second, and don't rotate your shoulders backward.

- This exercise has carryover effects for the High Pull because it represents a subset of that exercise's full range of motion.

Shrugs, One-Arm

Develops the trapezius muscles.

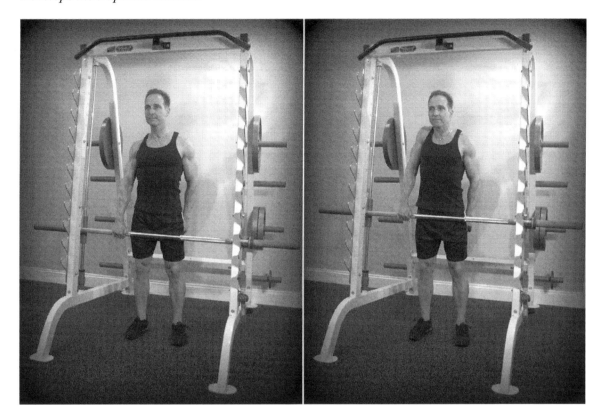

This unilateral version of the traditional shrug increases the intensity of the movement.

Performance

While standing, hold the Smith Machine bar in front of you with one arm using an overhand grip. Keep your arm straight and raise your shoulder as high as possible. Hold for a second and slowly lower to the starting position.

Tips & Technique

- Don't forget the key points of shrugging—keep your arm straight, use a full range of motion, hold the contraction at the top for a second, and don't rotate your shoulder backward.

- This is a useful movement if rehabilitating a shoulder injury because it helps you isolate the work to one side of the body.

Shrugs, Behind the Back

Develops the trapezius muscles.

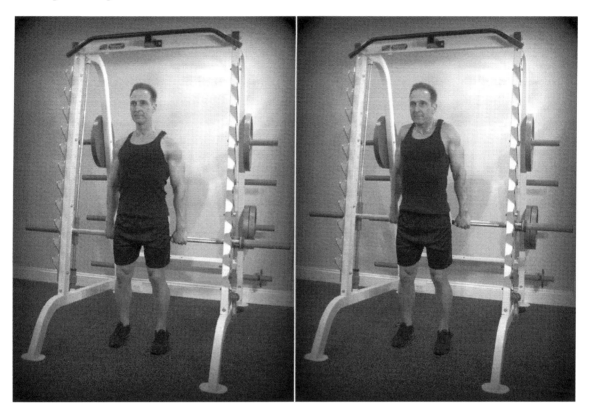

Performance

While standing, hold the Smith Machine bar behind you with an overhand grip. Keep your arms straight and raise your shoulders as high as possible. Hold for a second and slowly lower to the starting position.

Variations

One-Arm Shrugs Behind the Back

The one-arm version is useful for both corrective action and rehab. As always, unilateral movements increase the intensity of stress delivered to the target area as well as sharpen mental acuity.

Tips & Technique

- Don't forget the key points of shrugging—keep your arms straight, use a full range of motion, hold the contraction at the top for a second, and don't rotate your shoulders backward.

- Ensure your arms remain straight when performing this exercise. Bending your arms, even a little, starts to migrate this exercise into a hybrid of a shrug and an upright row behind the back.

- You won't be able to use as much weight in this movement as the traditional shrug. However, this version tends to help the novice learn and pattern the full height possibilities of a general shrug movement. I've witnessed countless beginners who think they are raising their shoulders as high as possible with the standard shrug, and then have them switch to this version and watch them discover new untapped limits of height.

Supported Shrugs

Develops the lower trapezius and mid-back.

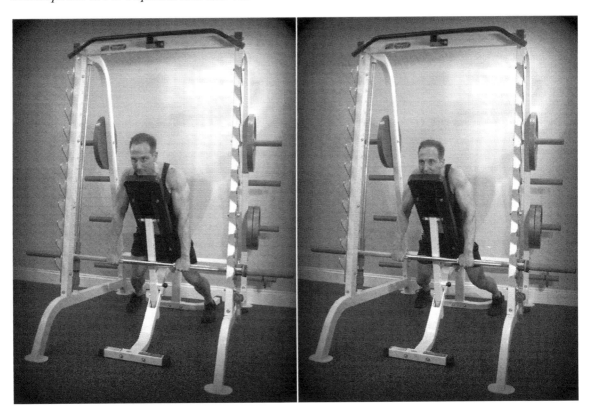

This version of the shrug provides an alternative for those experiencing temporary low back issues or for targeting the lower two trapezius muscles in the mid-back.

Performance

Set the Smith Machine bar to the lowest position. Place an incline bench, adjusted to about a 45-degree incline, just behind the bar so the seat is facing toward the rear of the machine (see the picture above for correct placement). Lie on the bench with your chest on the incline portion and hold the bar at shoulder width with an overhand grip. Keep your arms straight and raise your shoulders as high as possible. Hold for a second and slowly lower to the starting position.

Variations

One-Arm Supported Shrugs
The one-arm version is useful for both corrective action and rehab. As always, unilateral movements increase the intensity of stress delivered to the target area as well as sharpen mental acuity.

Tips & Technique

- You can adjust the bench angle to place more or less stress on the upper and lower trapezius muscles. A low angle turns this exercise into a general restricted range back rowing movement. As the angle increases, the involvement of the entire trapezius group increases.

- Don't forget the key points of shrugging—keep your arms straight, use a full range of motion, hold the contraction at the top for a second, and don't rotate your shoulders backward.

- If performed correctly, you should feel a pump and accumulating fatigue in your lower trap/mid-back area. If not, check your form and angle of incline.

Seated Shrugs

Develops the trapezius muscles.

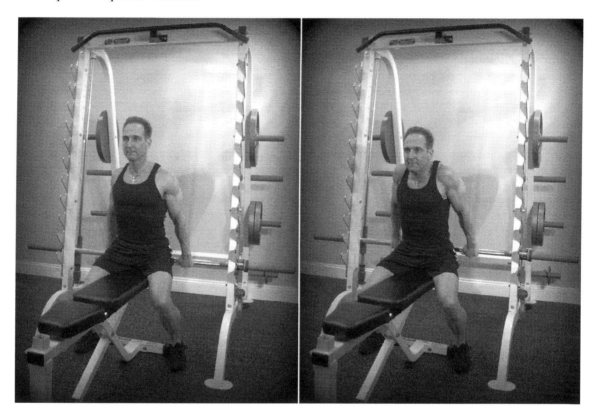

This version of the shrug reduces the compressive forces on the lower back and is an alternative for those experiencing this type of issue.

Performance

Set the Smith Machine bar at the lowest position. Place an exercise bench in front of the bar. While sitting on the back of the bench, hold the bar with a shoulder width overhand grip and raise your shoulders as high as possible. Hold for a second and slowly lower until the bar is hanging down as far as possible.

Variations

One-Arm Seated Shrugs
The one-arm version is useful for corrective action, rehab, increased intensity and focus.

Tips & Technique

- Keep your back straight when performing this exercise. Leaning forward or back may cause low back strain or impingement.

- Don't forget the key points of shrugging—keep your arms straight, use a full range of motion, hold the contraction at the top for a second, and don't rotate your shoulders backward.

Upright Rows

Develops the trapezius and the front and side deltoids, and creates separation between the deltoids and pectorals.

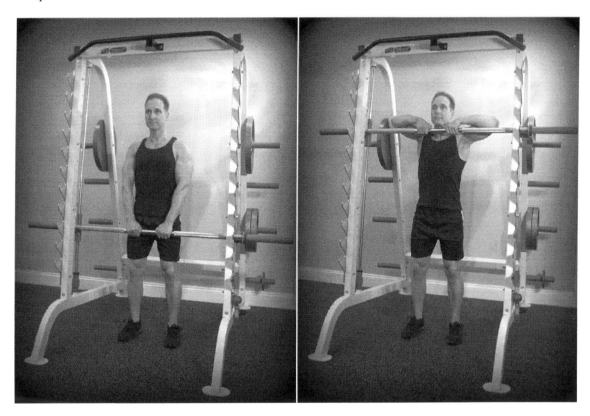

Upright rows are a transitional movement for the front of the shoulders, upper chest, traps and mid-back. In short, they work most of the upper extremities through a pulling action.

Performance

While standing, hold the Smith Machine bar in front of you with an overhand grip at shoulder width or slightly narrower. Pull the bar straight up, keeping it close to your body, until the bar is above the mid-point of your chest (good) or just under your chin (great). Slowly lower to the starting position.

Variations

One-Arm Upright Rows
If you are strong enough to perform this one-arm movement, it's an effective variation to increase

the intensity and check the relative symmetry of your strength. Make sure your elbow points directly out to your side throughout the movement.

Tips & Technique

- Keep your chest up, shoulders back and the bar close to your body for optimal performance and safety.

- As Goldilocks would relate, grip width is important here. Grips that are too narrow may impinge the wrists and shoulders of some, whereas grips too wide turn this into Wide-Grip Upright Rows, an entirely different exercise which targets the sides of the shoulders. A grip which is neither too wide, nor too narrow should be just right for most.

- A good mental cue is to think *"elbows up"*. Your elbows should be leading the charge upward, just slightly higher than your wrists and hands.

- For those with good shoulder flexibility, try to raise the bar up to the bottom of your chin—this should put your upper arms parallel with the floor. I don't recommend going any higher than this, because anatomical studies have shown greater probability of shoulder impingement occurring when pulling to excessive height.

Upright Rows, Behind the Back

Develops the trapezius.

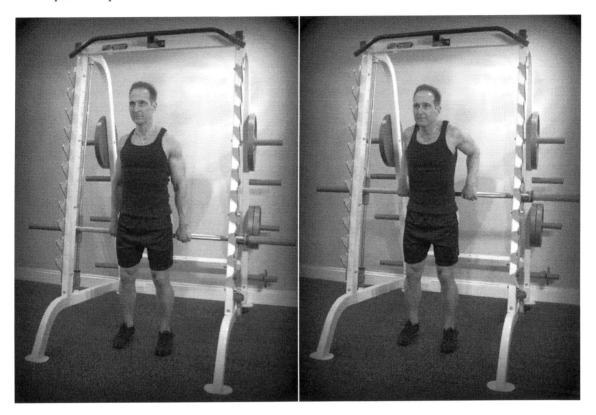

By moving the bar behind you, this version of the upright row targets the trapezius muscles and activates the biceps, while removing the stress on the front shoulders and upper chest.

Performance

While standing, hold the Smith Machine bar directly behind you with an overhand grip about shoulder width apart. Lift the bar as far up your back as possible, and then squeeze the muscles in your back. Slowly lower to the starting position.

Variations

One-Arm Upright Rows Behind the Back

The one-arm version is useful for both corrective action and rehab. As you know by now, unilateral movements increase the intensity of stress delivered to the target area as well as providing increased mental acuity.

Tips & Technique

- Although relatively unseen in most gyms, this was a favorite exercise of 8-time Mr. Olympia Lee Haney. Performed correctly, you should feel all the muscles contracting in your mid-back (that's the two lower trapezius muscles). Think about trying to make yourself as narrow as possible as you raise the bar—your cue is *"narrow and high"*.

- This exercise works well in combination with the traditional upright row. Many of the assistive muscles that get worked in the upright row (shoulders, upper chest) get stretched in this version. Try performing a few sets of this exercise after you've completed your regular upright row work or consider super-setting the two by performing one followed immediately by the other.

- Due to mechanical and leverage limitations here, you won't be able to use nearly as much weight as you can with regular upright rows—but that's not the point. Pulling the bar as high up your back and holding the contraction for a second will uncover the gold in this exercise.

High Pulls

Develops the trapezius, shoulders and upper back.

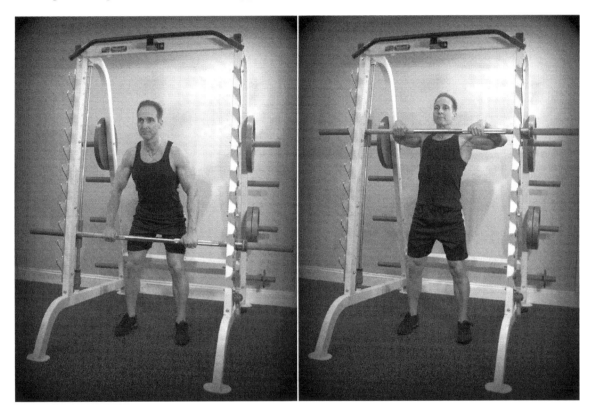

Performance

Stand with your feet about shoulder width apart. Bend your knees and hips so the bar touches the mid-thigh and hold the bar with an overhand grip a little wider than shoulder width apart. Your back and arms should be straight. From this position, pull the weight up explosively, shrugging your shoulders as you extend the hips and straighten your legs. Once you are fully upright, continue to pull the bar by bending your elbows out to the sides and lifting the bar as high as possible. Slowly lower the weight and repeat.

Tips & Technique

- Make no mistake—this is an explosive power movement which engages both lower and upper body, so you should be able to use some heavy weight on this exercise—heavier than you can use with Upright Rows. Performed correctly, High Pulls can add more muscle on your shoulder, trap and upper back structure than most other exercises. For this reason, the free weight version is a favorite of Olympic lifters, powerlifters and strongmen worldwide.

- You can start this exercise with the bar positioned near the floor (traditional High Pulls) or with the bar near the lower thighs (Hang Pulls). The picture above illustrates the Hang Pull, because that particular Smith Machine does not allow the bar to rest near the floor.

- A perfectly performed High Pull is a seamless movement—your heels should rise off the floor as the power of your hip and knee extension, coupled with the shrug and pull, send the bar skyward. Visualize an Apollo rocket taking off, with you as the booster engine. You should be attempting to accelerate the bar throughout the movement. Think *acceleration*.

Triceps

When someone asks you to show them a muscle, it's a universal call to arms—arms everywhere rise up and flex to proclaim to the world how big (or small) your biceps are. However, if you are concerned with proportionate strength and muscular development, as well as aesthetics, when that arm goes up, their eyes should be drawn slightly down from the bicep, as their mouths hang agape to behold that hardened mass on the lower (backside) part of your upper arm. That's because, regardless of race, creed or religion, you're a human, and two-thirds of your upper arm mass is pure triceps.

Because the primary purpose of the triceps is to straighten the arms, all triceps work boils down to pushing/extension movements, such as dips, presses, pushdowns and extensions. Although you can't perform pushdowns on a Smith Machine, you can perform presses, dips and extensions to fully develop your triceps.

The extensions deserve a special note here. Free weight extensions, performed with a barbell or dumbbell(s), use an arcing motion, so what we are limited to on a Smith Machine is a faux extension, using explicit body positioning in relation to the bar path in order to maximize the triceps stress along that linear path. Not as good as the free weight version, but it will get most of the job done if that's all you have to work with.

Here are the important points for working your triceps effectively:

- For packing pure muscle mass onto the triceps, there are no equivalents to close-grip bench presses and dips. It's no surprise that both are multi-joint movements.

- For maximal development of the long-head of the triceps (the biggest triceps muscle and the biggest muscle of the upper arm—comprising about 50% of your total upper arm size), seated or standing extensions with your elbows pointing straight up are what you want. This places the long-head into a pre-stretched position, requiring it to travel across the full range of motion until the arm is completely straight. That equates to maximum development. Don't sacrifice weight for form on these exercises. Smart bodybuilders use this simple science to great effect in building outrageously sized upper arms.

- When performing any type of triceps exercise, don't accelerate your arms into a straightened position—this will cause all kinds of elbow issues as you age. You want to decelerate just as you reach full contraction, and then squeeze the triceps as hard as possible.

Here are the Smith Machine exercises to work your triceps:

- Close-Grip Bench Press
- Reverse-Grip Bench Press
- Dips, Behind the Back
- Extensions, Fixed Bar
- Extensions, Lying
- Extensions, Seated
- Extensions, Standing

Close-Grip Bench Press

Develops the overall triceps.

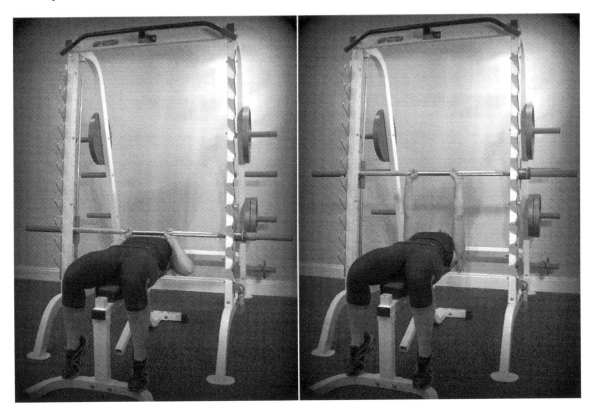

This is the most effective triceps exercise you can perform on the Smith Machine.

Performance

Place a bench under the Smith Machine bar. Set the safeties just above the height of the bench. Lie on the bench, hold the bar with your hands about 12-14" apart and unhook the bar. Lower the bar slowly until it just touches your mid-chest. Keep the elbows close to your body and press the bar upward until your arms are locked out.

Variations

Incline & Decline Close-Grip Bench Presses
Although the traditional flat bench version of this exercise is most common, the incline variation is great for building the upper/inner chest, as well as the triceps. The decline version introduces a

shorter range of motion and a more favorable leverage angle, allowing you to use heavier weights—something occasionally useful for powering past plateaus.

Tips & Technique

- Using a narrow grip on presses changes the emphasis primarily from the chest to the triceps.

- Contrary to popular belief, using a close-grip on these presses doesn't mean your hands grip the bar a couple inches apart. Try that with heavy weights and your wrists will start screaming at you. MRI scans of individuals performing this exercise have shown that hand spacing as wide as 12-14 inches apart creates the same amount of triceps involvement as grip widths half that distance. Stick with placing your hands about a foot apart on this exercise and you'll be good to go from beginner to world-class presser.

- Common mistakes with this exercise include incorrect hand spacing (too wide or too close), flaring the elbows out, bouncing the bar off the chest, lowering the bar too low or high on the torso, arching of the back, and not keeping a stable base with your feet. Try to keep your elbows as close to the body as possible. The bar should be lowered to mid-chest. Keep your feet flat on the floor. Don't lift your heels—this tends to assist with excessive back arching, shifting the stress to the front shoulders.

- You can increase the intensity of this exercise by intentionally not locking out your elbows at the top of the movement, keeping continuous tension on the triceps. Because lockout movements are an important concept in any type of weight training, alternating workouts between lockout and continuous tension presses is a good strategy for overall effectiveness on this exercise.

- Partial reps work wonderfully as part of an overall strength strategy—notice I said "as part of", and not "exclusively". Additionally, Drop Sets are an effective technique here as well. I encourage you to explore both.

Reverse-Grip Bench Press

Develops the triceps and the chest.

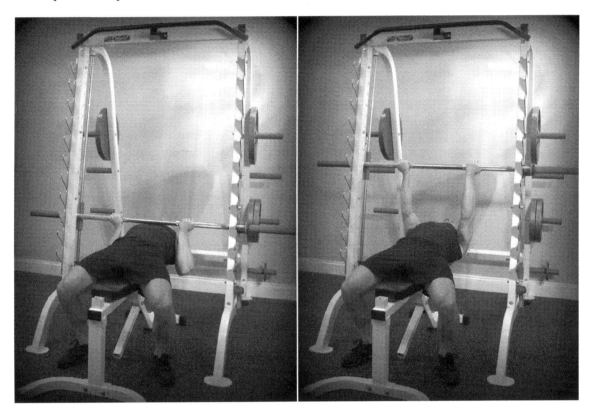

Performance

Place a bench under the Smith Machine bar. Set the safeties just above the height of the bench. Lie on the bench and hold the bar with an underhand grip about shoulder width apart. Unhook the bar and lower it slowly until the bar just touches your lower chest. Keep the elbows close to your body and press the bar up until your arms are locked out.

Tips & Technique

- You rarely see this exercise performed anymore. Why?—because it's like going on a first date. At first, it's awkward and clumsy, then after spending some time together you either decide to continue or it just doesn't feel right and you go back to your old standby.

- Make sure to wrap your fingers and thumb tightly around the bar. In general, it's always good to grip the bar tightly regardless of the exercise, but on this one it really helps get you acquainted and off to a promising future. This is not the exercise to experiment with a faux (thumb-less) grip, fashionable in bodybuilding circles.

- Common mistakes with this exercise include incorrect hand spacing (too wide or too close), flaring the elbows out, bouncing the bar off the chest, lowering the bar too low or high on the torso, arching of the back, and not keeping a stable base with your feet. Try to keep your elbows as close to the body as possible. The bar should be lowered to mid-chest. Keep your feet flat on the floor. Don't lift your heels—this tends to assist with excessive back arching, shifting the stress to the front shoulders.

- You can increase the intensity of this exercise by intentionally not locking out your elbows at the top of the movement, keeping continuous tension on the triceps. Because lockout movements are an important concept in any type of weight training, alternating workouts between lockout and continuous tension presses is a good strategy for overall effectiveness on this exercise.

- Partial reps work wonderfully as part of an overall strength strategy—notice I said "as part of", and not "exclusively". Additionally, Drop Sets are an effective technique here as well. I encourage you to explore both.

Dips, Behind the Back

Develops the thickness of the triceps, especially around the elbow.

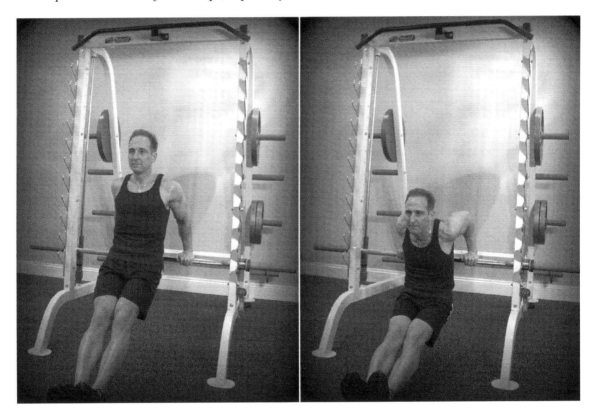

Performance

Set the height of the Smith Machine bar at about knee height and lock the safeties to keep it there. Grip the bar slightly wider than shoulder width behind you, place your heels on the ground out in front of you and bend your arms, slowly lowering your body until your upper arms are parallel with the floor or you feel a slight stretch in the chest or shoulders. Straighten the arms to return to the starting position.

Variations

Elevated Dips Behind the Back
To make this exercise more challenging, elevate your feet on an exercise bench.

Tips & Technique

- Don't be misled here—these are not your standard triceps dips using dedicated thick-handled dipping bars. That exercise is one of the kings of triceps builders. Because the Smith Machine doesn't have dipping bars, you'll have to use this alternate form of dips instead using body weight and perhaps an elevated bench. Not as efficient or effective, but will still get the job done.

- This exercise can help you slowly increase your shoulder flexibility over time (it also stretches the chest). Set the bar to the lowest position and work up from there. For those with pre-existing shoulder issues, avoid this exercise. Typically, you want to lower yourself until your upper arms are parallel with the floor. Descending below parallel brings the chest and shoulders increasingly into play.

- You can increase the intensity of this exercise by intentionally not locking out your elbows at the top of the movement, keeping continuous tension on the triceps. Because lockout movements are an important concept in any type of weight training, alternating workouts between lockout and continuous tension dips is a good strategy for overall effectiveness on this exercise.

- You can also decrease the intensity of the exercise by placing your feet closer towards your torso, by bending your knees. Beginners who can't perform a full rep using the straight leg method should try this alternative. Advanced trainers can re-position their feet inward as their triceps fatigue, enabling them to continue the set in forced rep fashion.

- If the design of your Smith Machine permits, you can set the bar height so that your glutes just touch the floor at full dipping depth. This will allow you to continue performing reps until you reach complete failure, without fear of falling or hyperextending the shoulders.

Extensions, Fixed Bar

Fully stretches and develops the lower area of the triceps.

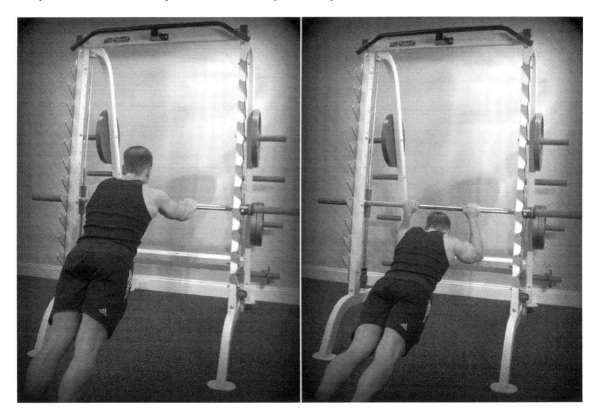

Performance

Lock the Smith Machine bar at about waist height and set the safeties to keep it there. While standing, bend forward at the waist and grip the bar about shoulder width apart. Making sure your elbows are locked, extend your feet behind you until you are in a push-up position with your entire body in a rigid line. Slowly lower your body so that your head travels under the bar by bending your arms—keep the body straight throughout. Return to the starting position by extending your arms.

Variations

Fixed Bar Close-Grip Pushups
This is a great variation to immediately switch to after your triceps become fatigued with the extensions. Because you'll be using a close-grip on the bar and pushing (like you are performing a Close-Grip Bench Press), this will activate the pectorals, allowing you to continue to exhaust the

triceps with assistance from the chest. It's also a good exercise to use if you can't perform full reps using the extension technique described above. Keep your body straight when performing this variation.

Tips & Technique

- If you don't have the strength (yet) to perform this exercise standing with a rigid body on your feet, you can kneel and perform it from your knees. This is an effective exercise that really stresses the long head of the triceps, stretching it all the way into the back of the shoulders. It's also just a damn good method for stretching the triceps at the end of an arm workout.

- You can increase or decrease the difficulty of this exercise by raising or lowering the height of the bar. Higher bar placements are easier to perform, whereas lower bar placements, below waist level, are much harder because full-body weight, physics and gravity conspire against you.

- Above all else, keep your body/torso straight throughout the movement.

Extensions, Lying

Works the triceps all the way from the elbow down to the lats.

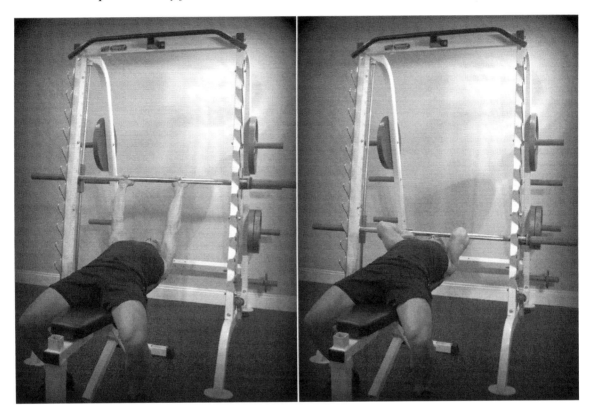

Performance

Place a bench under the Smith Machine bar and set the safeties above the height of the bench. Lie on the bench with your feet flat on the floor. Hold the bar with a narrow overhand grip, unlock the bar and extend your arms overhead. Keep your elbows stationary and lower the weight to your forehead. Return to the starting position by extending your arms. Try to keep your elbows as close to your body as possible.

Variations

Incline & Decline Extensions

This exercise can also be performed using incline and decline benches. Although the incline variation of this exercise reduces the overall range of motion by using a partial press movement pattern, it does allow you to use heavier weights—something you may want to consider in order to break past a plateau. Experiment with various levels of incline and decline here.

Tips & Technique

- Try using the same 12-14 inch hand spacing you used with the Close-Grip Bench Press.

- Although the free weight version of all extension exercises uses an arcing movement, you can still get most of the benefits with this linear variation. Just think of it as close-grip pressing to your head.

Extensions, Seated

Develops the inside and rear heads of the triceps.

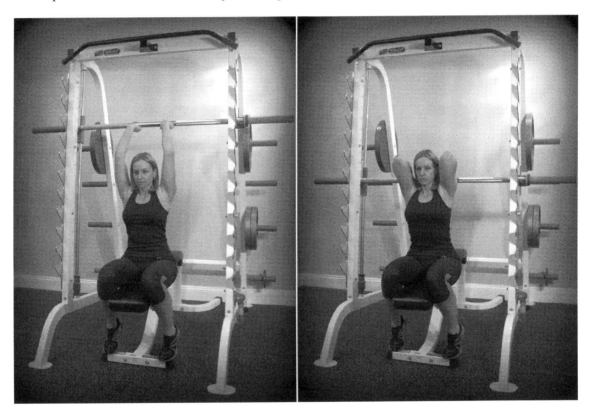

Performance

Place a bench under the Smith Machine bar and set the safeties to about chest level. Sit on the bench slightly in front of the bar with your feet flat on the floor. Hold the bar with a narrow grip, unlock the bar and extend your arms overhead. Keep your elbows stationary and lower the bar behind your head as far as possible. Return to the starting position by extending your arms.

Tips & Technique

- Any triceps exercise where your elbows point to the ceiling fully activates the long head of the triceps. If you want big triceps, that's your muscle because it comprises about half the size of your upper arm.

- Don't sacrifice form over weight here—keep your elbows as close to the sides of your head as possible.

Extensions, Standing

Develops the full sweep of the triceps.

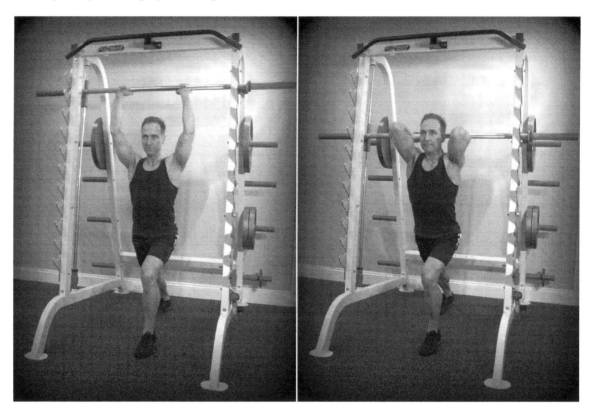

Performance

Set the Smith Machine safeties at about shoulder height. Stand slightly in front of the bar. Hold the bar with a shoulder-width grip, unlock the bar and extend your arms overhead. Keep your elbows stationary and lower the weight behind your head as far as possible. Return to the starting position by extending your arms.

Tips & Technique

- The standing version of this exercise allows you to incorporate some assistive cheating with your legs as your triceps begin to reach muscular failure. That equates to heavier weights and bigger arms. Just don't forget to balance the use of this version with the more strict seated variety for optimal results.

- You can stand with either the feet at shoulder width apart, or with one foot forward of the other (as pictured above). Try each type of stance and see which provides you with the most stability. As the weights increase on this exercise you may discover the offset stance provides a more stable base.

- Try to keep your elbows as close to the sides of your head as possible.

7

The Workouts

This section presents a plethora of workouts using the exercises described and depicted earlier. Use these as a basis for your workouts, depending on your goals, time, and availability of other workout equipment.

Sometimes, the realities of life dictate the types of workouts you can do. When you are in high school or college, maybe still living at home with your parents, with no spouse or kids to tend to, the boundaries are still wide. You can launch into those 1-2 hour workouts five or six days a week if you want to. For most of us though, intensive study at school, needing to stay late at work to meet that project deadline, or rushing home to grab a quick bite and get the girls to gymnastics practice takes precedent. The boundaries have moved inward. But don't despair, most of the types of workouts you can do are still very viable, given those constraints. Although you may not be able to do that six-day a week split bodybuilding routine anymore, it doesn't mean you can't get stronger, build more muscle, and lose more fat than ever before. The workouts in this section will show you how.

For example, if you are short on time but want to get in a whole body workout, try some of the circuit training workouts. If you need to improve a specific weak area of your body, try one of the weak point training workouts. If even more muscle mass is your thing or you've hit a plateau with your regular workout, look at the strength training and bodybuilding workouts. Finally, if you find yourself with an injury and are trying to rehab or work around the area, you might find some of the suggested workout accommodations in the injury rehab section worth considering. There is something for everyone, regardless of time, schedule, or situation.

One thing I want to mention right up front—all of the workouts listed below assume that you only have a Smith Machine available for your weight training efforts. If you have access to barbells, dumbbells, cables, kettlebells, tractor axles, logs, pipes, chains, or stones, then by all means feel free to substitute those implements for any of the exercises listed in each workout. In fact, I encourage it. However, if you're in an injured state, are a relative beginner who doesn't have access to free weights, or is a little apprehensive about such things, then the workouts below will get you further along on your journey and help you transition to the unbounded options of the free-weight world.

You might also note that many of these workouts are quite simple in design. If that confuses or bothers you, recall what the ancient Chinese book of sword-fighting (*The Art of Iaido*), and more recently, Malcolm Gladwell stressed in his book *Outliers*, regarding the 10,000 hour rule. If you want to become an expert in something, you're probably going to need to perform it about 10,000 times. It's a lot quicker to get to 10,000 with something simple versus complex, because fewer things can go wrong. Conversely, don't judge a training program or workout based on a single day's experience.

In general, the workouts are progressive. At first, I'll go easy on you and describe everything you need to do if you're a beginner. For those of you with more experience, things get a little harder and I'll be more abrupt. Now let's get the basics of weight training out of the way, so that you understand how to do all of the workouts.

The Basics of Weight Training

Years ago, a friend of mine was house sitting while his neighbor was away for the weekend. As an impending storm approached, Jim thought it was a good idea to move his friend's motorcycle from the driveway into the garage. I asked, "Do you know how to ride a motorcycle?" Jim waved me off. "It can't be that hard." Once in a while, you get that gut feeling that something is going to go wrong. This was one of those times. After Jim and the motorcycle ended up eight feet into the forsythia hedge on the side of the house, it was time for me to go.

What's the lesson here? If you've never performed progressive resistance weight training, you don't just plop yourself under a bar and start pressing. You at least need to learn the basics so you have some sense of what you are doing and what effect it is having.

Reps

When you perform any weight training movement, it has a starting position, a midpoint, and an ending position (typically back at the start). That's one repetition of the exercise. Because nobody, other than exercise physiology textbooks, uses that full term, it's a rep to us and the rest of the world. It's also our atomic unit, our heart and soul of weight training. Everything begins and ends with the rep—it defines us.

High Reps or Low Reps?

The quintessential question when performing a weight training exercise is, "how many reps should I do?"

The answer depends on what your goals are.

As a general reference, go with this:

- **1-5 reps = Muscular Strength**
- **6-12 reps = Muscular Size**
- **13+ reps = Muscular Endurance**

Of course, that's a pretty simple generalization of a spectrum of effect, but it represents a good basis to work from.

In general, lower reps (1-5) build strength, moderate reps (6-12) build muscle size, and higher reps (15+) build muscular endurance. However, these are not absolutes or mutually exclusive. You will build muscle mass by doing sets of 3-5 reps. You will get stronger by sticking with 6-8 reps. And you can build muscular endurance by quickly performing sets of 8 reps with short rest intervals. The time-tested lesson is the general effect of low reps will be greater strength, moderate reps will be muscle mass, and high reps will be endurance—but spillover effects can still apply. Keep that in mind as you go through the workouts.

There's one more thing I need to mention regarding the number of reps so that you are forewarned—the lower the reps and the greater the weight, the higher the risk potential for injury. That's why it's paramount to properly warm-up before starting a workout or an exercise. High reps can also cause injury as well—performing weight-bearing exercises for multiple reps causes your body to progressively fatigue, and as fatigue accumulates, the natural reaction of mind and body is to start looking for the exit sign—urging you to make the exercise easier by loosening your form. Be careful of this siren song. Proper form and warm-ups throughout your workout and weight training life will greatly reduce the probability of injury. It's like everything else in life—the greater the risk, the greater the potential return. Only you can strike the balance that best fits your situation and goals.

Rep Tempo & Performance

When you listen to music that you enjoy, it's contains an inherent tempo, a cadence of beats and rhythm that speak to you. It's no different with weight training. You can lift a weight quickly, slowly, or somewhere in between—likewise, for lowering the weight. Just as some thrash to speed metal and others swoon to waltzes, there are various camps and ideologies regarding the optimal rep tempo and performance. Many strength coaches advocate lifting a weight as fast as possible— the logic progressing that as the weight increases the speed of the bar will decrease, even as your explosive lifting effort remains constant. Others advocate the SuperSlow™ method, taking seemingly eons to lift the weight and perhaps even longer to lower it.

Keep yourself in a rep tempo state of mind. You'll need to find your own balance between these extremes (maybe at an extreme) based on your physical capabilities and goals. The more rapidly you lift a weight, the greater the plate force on your body's structures. That equates to a higher probability of injury, but also a greater opportunity to successfully lift heavier weights. Lifting slowly dramatically decreases the odds of injury (it doesn't necessarily indicate the intensity is any lower), but often at the expense of heavier loads. In general, for most exercises start out with a nice, common rep tempo of 1-2 seconds to lift the weight and 2-4 seconds to lower it. (The big, compound power moves will be on the lower end of those numbers.) Adjust from there as you see fit.

Whatever you do, do not throw weights. You lift weights. This means actually using your muscles to lift and lower the weight. Anybody can throw weights around using poor form and momentum. It takes courage to start with light weights, learn the movements properly, and then slowly increase the weight. Failure to learn how to do the movements properly builds an unstable foundation that amplifies problems later and lands you in the injury rehab section of this book.

To conclude, make sure you lift and lower the weight appropriately, deliberately and under control at all times.

Sets

When you perform a series of reps, then stop, that's a set. It's as simple as that. Most workouts prescribe a series of sets and reps, such as five sets of five reps (5x5), three sets of twelve, ten and eight reps (3 x 12,10,8), a range of reps across a number of sets (3 x 6-10) or a range of sets across a range of reps (1-3 x 6-10). Welcome to your new language.

One more thing—all of the workouts presented below only list "working sets", the sets you perform after any warm-ups that you need. They are the sets that count.

Resting Between Sets

Besides the question, "how many reps should I do?" the next one usually arrives right after the first set is complete. "How long should I rest before the next set?" The answer, like most other things, is "it depends". It depends on the type of training you are performing and its inherent purpose. As we move along the weight training continuum, strength training typically requires longer rest periods (2-5 minutes between sets), bodybuilding-type training a little less (1-3 minutes) and circuit training or cardio-based training practically none at all. Each of the workouts presented in subsequent sections will give you a guideline of how long you should rest between sets. There's one last thing to remember here—the shorter the rest period, the higher the intensity, all other things being equal.

Progressive Resistance

Gradually, as you are able to increase the weight you use or the number of reps you can perform on an exercise (linear progression), your body will compensate from this stress by growing bigger and stronger. This is progressive resistance and it's the bedrock of any weight training activity. Of course, this can't go on forever or we would all be bench pressing 800 pounds, deadlifting over a thousand and picking up our cars. So you have to learn other techniques to increase overload and stimulate adaptation. The section on intensity techniques will provide you with some methods that are particularly well-suited for use on the Smith Machine. In general, progressive resistance works best when you start conservatively and gradually add weight in small increments over time. This is not a sprint—you are attempting to build a foundation of muscle and strength that will last for decades. Eventually, this creeping incrementalism will propel you to previously unimaginable results, especially when you look back a few years later and can't believe how relatively weak you were at the genesis of your efforts.

Warming Up

Always warm up before starting any workout. Muscles don't react well to sudden surprises, especially with ungodly poundage. Many trainers like to warm up with a little (5-10 minutes) light cardio work. I like to warm up with weights, using full-body movements such as light squats, presses and deadlifts, moving rapidly from one movement to the other. A lightly loaded (or empty) bar is great for this. What this does is two things—it gets your entire body prepared for hard physical work via systemic blood flow and it reinforces the same basic human movements that you will be using in your workout.

Sit or Stand?

Many of the exercises and workouts call for either standing or sitting versions of the same basic movement. You may wonder is it "better" to sit or stand when performing these exercises. Because you activate more muscles when you stand (especially the core muscles around your midsection, including your lower back), the general rule is:

> **Sit if you must, otherwise stand if you can.**

Obviously, if you have lower back issues you should sit. Many of the workouts listed below do specify a seated position for some exercises—in these cases, particularly those in the circuit training section, sitting was selected versus standing in order to keep the flow and pace of the workout steady (remember our link between exercises, workouts, and musical symphonies), without having to constantly move or adjust an exercise bench under, then away from the Smith Machine as you progress through the workout. Staccato-like bursts and intermissions are fine for strength training, but not so much for the ballet of circuit training.

Wraps, Belts, and Straps

Do yourself a favor from the outset and don't use these implements of assistance as you learn the exercises. Belts, straps and wraps are like the yin and yang of weightlifting. For novices and just about anyone not engaged in advanced powerlifting activity, they only provide a crutch—a false hope that will dash dreams of greatness later. Let the lower back and forearms strengthen, as those knee and elbow ligaments learn to handle increasing loads. It will make you a better person at bending over, picking things up and holding onto them, as well as providing for a better quality of life.

For those in the intermediate to advanced stages of weight training, a belt can be a useful aid, especially with deadlifts, squats and overhead presses. The belt helps you set up a strong lumber and thoracic core, as your abs and spinal erectors engage with the tightness of the belt. Don't use a belt when you are curling, performing calf raises, etc. It adds nothing.

The conclusion on these implements—know when and how to use 'em.

Keep a Record of Your Progress

No one wants to do this one. Yeah, I know, you just want to get on with the workout and lift and not be bothered with writing things down. Let me tell you something. Writing things down is one of the keys to success in life.

In order to maximize your results, you must keep accurate records of what you did. Sure, you can remember how many reps you got with 225lbs on the bench last time, but what about the weight and rep scheme you were using 6-8 weeks ago with stiff-legged deadlifts? Probably not.

These records become a barometer of accomplishment and a roadmap for further progress, giving you a clear plan of action. You wouldn't embark on the longest trip of your life into uncharted territory if you didn't have a map. Hell, even Hansel and Gretel were smart enough to leave a record of where they were, even if those damn birds ate the map. We talked about this earlier. You need to know where you are now and where you've been, so you can determine where you need to go.

Convinced? OK. Get yourself one of those little spiral bound notebooks (the really small ones) and a pencil (pen if you're confident) so that you can shove the pencil/pen into the spiral binding while you carry the notebook around as you work out. If the notebook is as small as your phone, you'll take it with you. (Oh, and there are phone apps for recording this stuff, so you really have no excuse—but I prefer paper records and not the damnation of software upgrades and the ethereal termination of my records.)

Things you need to record—the name of the exercise, the weight used and the number of reps performed. Don't forget the date of the workout. That's it. A typical entry might look something like this:

7/9/2013

Bench Press: 135x10, 185x8x8x6

Incline DB Press: 50x10x10x10

Six months later, when you look back on your entry from July 9, 2013 you'll see that you did four sets on bench press, starting with ten reps at 135lbs and then going up to 185lbs for the remaining three sets, where you got eight reps on the first set, eight for the second, and then could only get six reps on that last set. Subsequently, on the incline dumbbell press you managed ten reps for all three sets. All of this tells you something. The volume of your chest workout was seven sets. The next time you do chest with this same workout you need to either get all three sets of 185lbs for eight reps or increase the weight slightly and try for three sets of six. Likewise, you may want to either increase the weight on the incline dumbbell presses or get at least one additional rep each set. No more guessing what it's going to take to force adaptation to occur.

Time Waits for No One

Because most of us live in the real world of busy schedules and life balances, we need to be aware of how much time we have to devote to our passions and goals. In that vein, each workout presented below provides an estimated amount of time it should take to complete using the suggested rest intervals. Use this guide to select the appropriate workout that matches your goal, based on the time you have available that day or week. Remember, shorter workouts don't necessarily equate to easier ones. Some of the shortest workouts are also some of the most intense and exhausting, so you'll need to take your current energy level into consideration. That's why I've tried to order the workouts by increasing intensity, which essentially categorizes into experience level. Beginning weight trainers just don't have the capacity (yet) to perform high-intensity workouts.

Strength Training

Walk into almost any gym, head to the free weight section, and wait for a guy to walk over to the bench press—and just watch. Most of the time, it goes down like this. One 45lb. plate on each side of the bar, guy does about ten reps. Then, another 25-pounder on each side. About 6-8 reps this time. Now, two 45lb. plates on each side. Maybe one or two decent reps, then the back starts arching excessively, the bar bounces off the chest at the bottom with the bar rising ever so slowly at an odd angle and you start to wonder if he is performing manual defibrillation. Two or three total "reps" with that weight. Maybe he'll perform one more set like that, for one or two reps this time. Then, off to the cable crossover machine. This continues every workout, every week—forever (or until the membership runs out, the kids start arriving, or football season commences). That, my friends, is not strength training, or any sensible weight-training program of any sort.

The purpose of strength training is to get stronger. Whether you want to get stronger in a particular muscle group or get stronger overall, it's all strength training.

To recap the earlier discussion, traditional strength training workouts are characterized by a few compound multi-joint movements (squats, deadlifts, rows, presses) using heavy weights, relatively few sets, and ample rest times (2-5 minutes) between those sets for recovery. The workouts are often brief, intense and taxing.

Keys to Strength Training

- Few exercises
- Compound, multi-joint movements
- Heavy weights
- 1-5 reps per set
- 2-5 minutes rest between sets
- Low volume, high-intensity
- Start conservatively, gradually increasing the weight in small increments

For improving overall strength, you need to concentrate on the big pulling, pushing and hinge movements—this means deadlifts, bench presses, overhead presses, and squats. (The deadlift is the best overall measure of absolute strength, whereas the bench press is a good barometer of upper body strength—likewise, the squat is the best indicator of lower body strength.) Above all else, you need to have an effective plan—because you are reading this book, you now have the plans.

Although there are a plethora of strength training systems and approaches in use today, a few approaches have worked for thousands of people over the past few decades. We'll concentrate on those programs. Because strength training workouts are not quick, hit-and-run affairs, you'll need about 30-60 minutes to complete each workout in this section.

5x5 Programs (3 Days per Week)

Some of the oldest and most proven programs for increasing strength through weightlifting center on the concept of linear progression, using five sets of five reps (5x5) using basic compound movements.

There are three general protocols for performing 5x5 programs—the constant, ascending and descending weight methods.

Constant Weight Method

In the 5x5 constant weight method you use the same working weight for all five sets. Typically what this means is that you won't get all five reps on each set—in fact, you'll probably get less reps as you reach that fifth set. That's ok. What you want to focus on is eventually getting to that magical 25-rep total for all five sets. If your rep total goes up from workout to workout, you're getting stronger. Get to 25 and increase the weight for the next workout. That's linear progression. Then repeat the process.

So, what happens if your total goes down from the previous workout? Try again the next workout. Maybe you had a bad day, didn't get enough food or sleep, or maybe your rest periods between sets were too short. Make sure you use a consistent rest time between sets—otherwise, you're changing two variables at once, and we all know how much we like to solve quadratic equations. Look at the clock or get yourself a watch.

Ascending Weight Method

Not surprisingly, with this 5x5 method, after a few light warm-ups, gradually increase the weight on each of the five sets making sure to get five reps each time. The key here is determining how much to increase the weight for each set—you want to increase it as much as possible, without missing that fifth rep.

Descending Weight Method

This approach might not be so obvious. After a few warm-up sets (that don't count as part of your five working sets), go right to the heaviest weight you can handle for five reps. You need to find that weight that you can't get six reps with, but one not so heavy that you only get four reps. With experience, and your consistent record-keeping, this should be relatively easy for you to nail. The real key is determining how much weight to take off the bar for each subsequent set, so that you get five reps each time. Maybe you had a good night's sleep, ate like a bear, your biorhythms are in harmony, and today's horoscope says "you will be purposeful of mind and body today". In that case, you might not need to reduce the weight at all. Otherwise, try to decrease the weight as little as possible—just make sure you get those five reps.

Regardless of which 5x5 protocol you choose, try experimenting with rest intervals of one to five minutes. Five-minute rest periods should give you plenty of time to recover for your next set, allowing the use of maximum weight. Shorter rest periods will tax your cardiovascular system, making it harder to retain the same weights you used with the five-minute rest periods. But it's a good test—once in a while, try reducing your rest periods using a weight scheme that you succeeded with using five minute rest periods. If you can still handle it, then your entire system is getting stronger.

A final note before we get into the specific 5x5 workouts. **Beginners to strength training should start with three sets of five reps for the first couple months**, until their muscular, nervous, and adaptive systems become accustomed to this type of work.

Here are the strength training programs that we will examine.

- Basic A/B 5x5 Program
- Classic 5x5 Program ("The Big 3")
- Classic 5x5 Variation
- One-Lift Per Week 5x5 Program
- Variable Sequence 5x5 Program
- Higher Volume 5x5 Program

Basic A/B 5x5 Program

Workout time: 30-60 minutes

It doesn't get much more basic than this. Performed properly, consistently and intensely, this program will increase your overall strength regardless of whether you are beginner or experienced.

Perform this workout three days per week, alternating between **Workout A** and **Workout B** (most opt for the Monday, Wednesday, Friday schedule, but any three non-consecutive days will work). For each exercise listed, perform five sets of five reps (remember, beginners should do three sets of five).

Workout A	Workout B
Squats	Stiff-Legged Deadlift
Bench Press	Military Press, Standing
Deadlifts	Calf Raises

Classic 5x5 Program ("The Big 3")

Workout time: 45-60 minutes

Originated by legendary Johns Hopkins University strength coach Bill Starr, and described in detail in his seminal book, *Only the Strongest Shall Survive: Strength Training for Football*. Starr introduced us to his Zeus, Poseidon and Hades of weight training—"The Big 3" (squats, bench press, cleans), advocating an ascending weight protocol using a heavy, light, and medium strategy for the three workout days, and you should follow suit.

Of course, Starr's original program included the Power Clean—however, this is one exercise that requires complete freedom of movement and can't be duplicated effectively on the Smith Machine. Starr admitted that cleans irritate the shoulders of some lifters—in these cases he advocates substituting the high pull, and we'll do the same here. Finally, Starr included two supplemental exercises on each day, for higher reps.

In Starr's program, the heavy day sets the pace and weights for the week. The light and moderate days are based on the accomplishments of the heavy day. You want to increase the weight on each set by five (high pulls, bench press) or ten (squats) pounds, making sure to get the five reps. On the light day, only go up to the weight you used on the third set of the heavy day. Likewise, on the moderate day, only go up to the weight you used on the fourth set of the heavy day. I told you that you need that notebook to write stuff down.

Try this program for 4-6 weeks and see how you fare.

MON (Heavy)		WED (Light)		FRI (Moderate)	
High Pulls	5x5	High Pulls	5x5	High Pulls	5x5
Bench Press	5x5	Bench Press	5x5	Bench Press	5x5
Squats	5x5	Squats	5x5	Squats	5x5
Dips, Behind the Back	2-3 x 10-12	Curls	2-3 x 8-10	Dips, Behind the Back	2-3 x 8-10
Sit-Ups	2-3 x 15-20	Hanging Leg Raises	2-3 x 15-20	Sit-Ups	2-3 x 15-20

Classic 5x5 Variations

Workout time: 45-60 minutes

Many variations of Bill Starr's classic Big 3 program have appeared over the years, replacing some exercises and expanding on the volume of work.

Here is a common variation, which advances the squat to the opening lift and replaces the High Pulls with the Bent-Over Row.

MON (Heavy)		WED (Light)		FRI (Moderate)	
Squats	5x5	Squats or Front Squats	5x5	Squats	5x5
Bench Press	5x5	Military Press, Standing	5x5	Bench Press	5x5
Bent-Over Rows	5x5	Deadlifts	5x5	Bent-Over Rows	5x5
Dips, Behind the Back	2-3 x 10-12	Curls	2-3 x 8-10	Dips, Behind the Back	2-3 x 10-12
Sit-Ups	2-3 x 15-20	Hanging Leg Raises	2-3 x 15-20	Sit-Ups	2-3 x 15-20

Here's another classic 5x5 variation, taken from the annals of powerlifting greats. You'll notice this routine cycles through variations of the big three lifts, as well as assistance exercises.

MON (Heavy)		WED (Light)		FRI (Moderate)	
Squats	5x5	Bench Squats	5x5	Front Squats	5x5
Bench Press	5x5	Guillotine Presses	5x5	Floor Presses	5x5
Sumo Deadlifts	5x5	Romanian Deadlifts	5x5	Deadlifts	5x5
Military Press, Standing	3x5	Military Press, Seated	3 x 6-8	Press Behind the Neck	3 x 8-10
Curls	2 x 8-10	Drag Curls	2 x 8-10	Curls	2 x 10-12
Extensions, Lying	2 x 8-10	Dips, Behind the Back	2 x 10-12	Extensions, Standing	2 x 8-10

One-Lift Per Week 5x5 Program

Workout time: 30-60 minutes

Here's a simple, yet effective, strength training program you can perform three days per week. It's based on the classic 5x5 program of squats, presses, and deadlifts, but moves each of those lifts to their own dedicated day (once per week) and adds in a few more assistance exercises on the third day. For those of you who have trouble recovering from the lifts within a 48 hour timeframe (us older folk) this may be a viable alternative.

MON		WED		FRI	
Squats	5x5	Bench Press	5x5	Deadlifts	5x5
Chins (any type)	4 x failure	High Pulls	4x6	Curls	4x6
Bent-Over Rows	4x8	Military Press, Standing	4x6	Dips, Behind the Back	4 x failure
				Wrist Curls, Behind the Back	3 x 15-20
				Reverse Wrist Curls	3 x 15-20

Variable Sequence 5x5 Programs

Workout time: 30-60 minutes

The purpose of this 5x5 program is to provide sequencing variety, ensuring that your strength on each exercise has an optimized chance of progressing—it's designed to keep your body guessing and progressing in four week increments.

Use the workout as listed for the first four weeks. After that, rotate each exercise to the next position within the workout. For example, the Monday workout for week five would start with Deadlift, and follow with Bench Press and Squat. Four weeks later, Squat would be first, followed by Deadlift and Bench Press.

After trying this program for the full twelve weeks as listed, experiment with longer or shorter week sequences. Try changing the exercise order after every week or two, or perhaps change it only after six weeks. Discover what works best for you.

Perform five sets of five reps for all exercises listed.

Weeks 1-4

MON		WED		FRI	
Bench Press	5x5	Bent-Over Rows	5x5	Squat	5x5
Squat	5x5	Military Press, Standing	5x5	Bench Press	5x5
Deadlift	5x5	Lunges	5x5	Deadlift	5x5

Weeks 5-8

MON		WED		FRI	
Squat	5x5	Military Press, Standing	5x5	Bench Press	5x5
Deadlift	5x5	Lunges	5x5	Deadlift	5x5
Bench Press	5x5	Bent-Over Rows	5x5	Squat	5x5

Weeks 9-12

MON		WED		FRI	
Deadlift	5x5	Lunges	5x5	Deadlift	5x5
Bench Press	5x5	Bent-Over Rows	5x5	Squat	5x5
Squat	5x5	Military Press, Standing	5x5	Bench Press	5x5

Higher Volume 5x5 Program

Workout time: 60 minutes

Here's another alternative 5x5 program that's been used for decades due to its effectiveness. Some regard the front squat as the superior athletic squatting movement, and this routine substitutes that lift for the back squat. Perform this routine three times per week, using heavy, light, and moderate days as defined by the Classic 5x5 Program.

Perform five sets of five reps for all exercises listed.

MON (Heavy)		WED (Light)		FRI (Moderate)	
Heavy Upright Rows	5x5	Heavy Upright Rows	5x5	Heavy Upright Rows	5x5
Military Press, Standing	5x5	Military Press, Standing	5x5	Military Press, Standing	5x5
Front Squats	5x5	Front Squats	5x5	Front Squats	5x5
Bench Press	5x5	Bench Press	5x5	Bench Press	5x5
Deadlift (any variation)	5x5	Deadlift		Deadlift	

Other Strength Training Strategies

Although you can strength train effectively for most of the year with just a handful of basic movements, eventually you'll need to take a break and try some new ideas and exercises. Here's some proven alternatives for just such times—feel free to substitute any exercise into these options.

- 5x5 Two Days per Week

- One Lift per Day

- One Type of Movement per Day

- Partial Rep Movements

5x5 Two Days per Week

Workout time: 45-60 minutes

If you are really squeezed for time and only have two days per week to get stronger, you can adapt the typical 3-day per week 5x5 program into a two day routine. Here's how.

Workout A	Workout B
Squats	Squats
Bench Press	Bench Press
Sumo Deadlifts	Deadlifts

You'll need at least two days of rest between each workout. Just remember, two training days per week is the bare minimum for eliciting strength gains. Anything less and you might as well take up bowling or golf instead.

One Lift per Day

Workout time: 30-60 minutes

The name says it all. Pick one exercise and do it for the entire workout, each set for 3-5 reps. Finish with a couple back-off sets of 10-12 reps. You'll be amazed at how this type of workout can clear and focus the mind. After you select your exercise for the day, there's really nothing else to think about, except maybe when to switch from the 3-5 reps to the finishing sets of 10-12 reps. With clarity of purpose, your efforts are laid bare. Don't give the workout your maximum effort, and the record will show it. Do and you might remember it for a long time.

Try a Push Day, a Pull Day, a Squat Day and even a Whole Body Day (Squat+Press) with this program.

Movement	Exercise (pick one)
Pull Day	Deadlifts
	Sumo Deadlifts
	Romanian Deadlifts
	Bent-Over Rows
Push Day	Bench Press
	Incline Press
	Decline Press
	Military Press
Squat Day	Squats
	Front Squats
Whole Body Day	Squats + Press Behind the Neck
	Overhead Squats + Push Press
	Overhead Squats + High Pulls

One Type of Movement per Day

Workout time: 30-60 minutes

Expanding on the one lift per day concept, you can schedule entire workout days dedicated to a specific type of movement—a push day, a pulling day, and a leg day, using multiple exercises. In addition, unchain yourself from 5x5 and try three sets of eight reps for each exercise, with only a one-minute rest between sets. The next week, reacquaint yourself with 5x5—keep alternating the weekly set/rep scheme to keep the adaptation occurring.

DAY 1 (Pushing)		DAY 2 (Legs)		Day 3 (Pulling)	
Military Press, Seated	3x8 or 5x5	Front Squats	3x8 or 5x5	Deadlifts	3x8 or 5x5
Bench Press	3x8 or 5x5	Overhead Squats	3x8 or 5x5	Bent-Over Rows	3x8 or 5x5

Partial Rep Movements

Eventually, the linear progress will stop. Before the grief, agony and thoughts of hanging it all up set in, consider why you can't increase the weight anymore. More than likely you can get the weight moving at the start, and find it easier at the end of the movement, but have a hell of a time in that middle range. Maybe it just won't move after three reps or you can't seem to finish the press at the top.

You've discovered a sticking point—a place in the range of motion in a particular exercise where things get real tough. Several reasons can cause this, such as failure to follow the workout correctly or consistently, improper or inadequate nutrition, insufficient rest, lack of change, and gravity.

At times like this, the last thing you want to do is keep doing the same thing you've already done, expecting the results to change. In case you didn't know, that's the clinical definition of insanity.

However, there are lots of things you can do at this point, most of them maybe not so obvious (train more consistently, eat better, get more sleep and worry less) and some of them staring you right in the face from an earlier chapter. We're talking about employing exercises which use a limited range of motion. Often, consistent use of limited range exercises with increasing weights will allow you to return to the full range exercise and blast right past those plateaus.

The great thing about power racks and Smith Machines are that you can position the bar to start at the exact point where you begin having trouble and work on that area.

Here's some examples of partial range exercises you can use when you get stuck—but remember, you have a Smith Machine, so you can do this with any exercise.

Issue	Partial Rep Resolution
Deadlift is Stuck	Try Rack Pulls or Sumo Deadlifts
Bench Press is Stuck	Try Floor Presses
Straight-Leg or Stiff-Legged Deadlift is Stuck	Try Romanian Deadlifts
Military Press is Stuck	Try Push Presses
Upright Rows are Stuck	Try High Pulls

What you want to do is start at a dead stop at the precise sticking point location for sets of 3-5 reps. Think of each rep as its own mini-set, where you reset from a complete stop each time—no bar bouncing here, please. This strategy is particularly effective for presses and deadlifts.

◆ ◆ ◆ ◆

So, after you've given one or two of these strength training programs a serious, sustained effort, how strong are you now? If you've been recording your progress, you have your answer. You know your starting numbers and your current levels, so it should be easy to gauge just how much stronger you are now. If you haven't been recording your progress, then how the hell do you know where you've been, where you are, and where you need to go? More than likely, you're lost.

What about long-term goals?

Your goal here should be to get as strong as you can. Only you will discover those personal limits—which you probably don't know or can't even imagine yet. In the meantime, strive for a deadlift double your body weight, a body weight bench press, and perhaps an overhead press as close to your weight as possible. Then go beyond.

Bodybuilding

The first time I walked into the gym and saw Nathan I couldn't help but stare. This guy was in his late thirties, about 5'8" and 200 pounds, every muscle perfectly developed and lean as hell. Although he looked like you could bleed him out with a paper cut, his muscle density looked puncture-proof. I walked over and said, "How long have you been bodybuilding?"

"Don't ever call me a bodybuilder again. I'm a powerlifter."

Yes, he was—and a good one at that. The records of his regional contest accomplishments in issue after issue of *Powerlifting USA* verified it. Five hundred pound squats and deadlifts. Three hundred pound bench presses. For the remainder of the years I trained at that gym, all I ever saw him do were heavy squats, deadlifts, and presses of various sorts, for five sets of five reps, evoking images of the legendary Reg Park. Throw in some weighted sit-ups at the end of the workout. No deviations—ever.

My point is do you get the point by now? Strength training builds strength, and it builds muscle, lots of muscle. Of course, genetics and diet often dictates how all that turns out. Every wannabe bodybuilder started life as a strength trainer, using simple linear progression methods as Nathan used.

Starting the journey is one thing, but continuing on the path for sustained periods is another. For most, strength training is monotonously boring, due to the extreme non-variety of exercises. This is one of the main reasons you don't see a whole bunch of massively muscled and exceptionally strong people walking around. It requires extreme perseverance and a limited focus. In today's fast-paced, Internet-driven, I want it now world, most people don't spend enough time building that base of strength and muscle mass, opting to migrate all too quickly for the cable crossover and the preacher curls. They quickly end up in the high-volume world of hypertrophy-based bodybuilding training.

Regardless how you arrived here or how long it took, the purpose of bodybuilding training is to add as much symmetrical, lean muscle growth to your physique as your goals and genetics dictate. The bodybuilders of the past century have established two distinct training philosophies based around volume and intensity to accomplish this:

Low-volume, High intensity

This approach has you performing few working sets, but at a high-intensity, not unlike the strength training workouts you just read about. The difference here is the expansion of the variety of exercises used (both compound and isolation), with a slightly higher rep range (6-8). Typically, you take each working set to complete muscular failure (that's the intensity part of the equation). Aim for about six working sets for smaller muscle groups (arms, calves, and abs) and about eight sets for larger ones (chest, back, shoulders, and legs). If you are like most people, you lead a busy life of work and family and probably don't like to waste things, like time. This is a good way to train if you are consistently limited by time.

High-volume, Lower intensity

If you've ever thumbed through any of the popular muscle magazines, this is the type of training they contain and endorse, almost exclusively. Long workouts with lots of sets, and reps. These volume-based workouts are great for people with good to great recovery ability (late teens to early 30s), favorable genetics (mesomorphs or endo-mesomorphs), and those using performance-enhancing drugs. For individuals with ample workout time meeting those criteria, this is a good option. Lastly, note that I am specifying 'lower intensity' workouts here and not 'low intensity'. There is a difference.

I recommend you try both high-intensity and high-volume approaches each for 6-8 weeks and determine which suits you best. Some people thrive on high-intensity training, whereas others proceed better on higher volume. Allow your body to dictate the path. Perhaps the optimal strategy is to alternate the use of each method for 6-8 week cycles. This tends to keep the body adapting and free of injury—not to mention keeping your enthusiasm high and your sanity in check, which is always good for overall health and fitness longevity. Finally, relax—there's no one true path to success in any weight training endeavor, and the sooner you come to grips with that, the quicker you'll get down the road.

Keys to Bodybuilding

- An expanded repertoire of exercises
- Compound, multi-joint movements combined with isolation exercises
- Moderate to heavy weights
- 6-12 reps per set
- 1-2 minutes rest between sets
- Low volume/high-intensity or high volume/lower intensity

Like the strength trainer, for packing on lots of muscle mass, we want to concentrate first on compound, multi-joint movements for large muscle groups—think chest, back, and thighs. Consistent, heavy weight targeted at these areas will thicken your overall musculature like nothing else. Like the sculptor beginning a new project, this strategy will add slabs of raw muscle to your physique, while the isolation exercises act as the refining chisel. Always try to keep the isolation exercises—the great differentiator between strength athletes and bodybuilders—as the secondary component of your overall bodybuilding plan.

From the overall collection of exercises presented earlier, here's the shortened list of compound, multi-joint exercises for the large muscle groups that are central to building muscle mass:

Muscle Group	Mass Building Exercises
Chest	Bench Press
	Incline Press
	Decline Press
	Floor Press
Back	Deadlifts
	Partial Deadlifts ("Rack Pulls")
	Sumo Deadlifts
	Bent-Over Rows
	Chins, To the Front
	Chins, Behind the Neck, Wide-Grip
	Chins, Close-Grip
	Good Mornings
	Pull-Ups
Thighs (Quads)	Squats
	Front Squats
	Bench Squats
	Bench Front Squats
	Half Squats
Hamstrings	Romanian Deadlifts
	Stiff-Legged Deadlifts
Shoulders	Military Press, Standing
	Military Press, Seated
	Push Press
	Heavy Upright Rows

Muscle Group	Mass Building Exercises
Traps	Shrugs
	Upright Rows
	High Pulls
Biceps	Close-Grip Pull-Ups
Triceps	Close-Grip Bench Press
	Dips, Behind the Back

All of these exercises form the nexus of our bodybuilding workouts. Now, let's start examining some classic bodybuilding full-body workouts.

Full Body Workouts

These workouts pack on muscle over your whole body—therefore, perform these workouts three times per week, scheduling a day of rest between each. Monday, Wednesday, Friday or Tuesday, Thursday and Saturday are popular scheduling approaches here.

For those transitioning from pure strength-training workouts to bodybuilding-oriented, hypertrophy-based workouts, start with one of the transitional workouts described below. If you're not arriving from a strength-base (and why not?), evaluate your level of experience and select an appropriate workout, based on that experience and available time.

- Workout #1: 15-30 minutes

- Workout #2: 20-40 minutes

- Workout #3: 20-60 minutes

- Workout #4: 30-60 minutes

- Workout #5: 30-45 minutes

- Workout #6: 30-45 minutes

- Workout #7: 20-60 minutes

- Workout #8: 30-45 minutes

- Workout #9: 30-45 minutes

- Workout #10: 30-60 minutes

- 4-Month Program: 45-60 minutes

- Full-Body to Split-Body Program: 20-60 minutes

Bodybuilding: Full-Body Workout #1

Workout time: 15-30 minutes

If you are transitioning from pure strength training workouts to bodybuilding-style workouts, this is a great routine to start with, because it contains many familiar strength training exercises—however, here the rep range is higher. For this full body workout, alternate between **Workout A** and **Workout B** each workout day. Complete 1-3 sets of each exercise for 6-10 reps on upper body exercises, and 10-20 reps on lower body exercises. Take 1-2 minutes rest between sets. Perform this workout three days per week. Suggested workout days are Monday, Wednesday and Friday, although you can alter that to anything that fits your schedule—just make sure to keep one rest day between each workout.

Workout A		Workout B	
Squats	1-3 x 10-20	Deadlift	1-3 x 6-10
Dips, Behind the Back	1-3 x 6-10	Bench Press or Incline Press	1-3 x 6-10
Bent-Over Row	1-3 x 6-10	Chins (any type)	1-3 x 6-10
Crunches	1-3 x failure	Hanging Leg Raises, Bent-Knee	1-3 x failure

Bodybuilding: Full-Body Workout #2

Workout time: 20-40 minutes

This is another good workout for those transitioning from strength training to bodybuilding. Perform this workout three times per week, with a day of rest between each. Complete three sets of 8, 6, and 4 reps for each exercise (be sure to warm-up on each exercise). Take 1-3 minutes rest between sets. When you are able to get all 18 total reps for the 3 sets on any exercise, add a little more weight the next workout.

3 Days per Week	
Heavy Upright Rows	3 x 8, 6, 4
Military Press, Standing	3 x 8, 6, 4
Front Squats	3 x 8, 6, 4
Bench Press	3 x 8, 6, 4
Crunches	1 x failure

Bodybuilding: Full-Body Workout #3

Workout time: 20-60 minutes

This transitional workout introduces some new exercises, increases the reps, and decreases the rest intervals. Do this workout three times per week, with a day of rest between each. Start with three sets per exercise and each week add another set until you are performing five sets per exercise by the third week. Take 1-2 minutes rest between sets. Your body has no choice but to adapt.

3 Days per Week	
Squats	3-5 x 10
Push-Ups	3-5 x 10
Chin-Ups (any type):	3-5 x 10
Crunches or Leg Raises	1 x failure

Bodybuilding: Full-Body Workout #4

Workout time: 30-60 minutes

This is a complete hypertrophy-based program that requires three days per week, 30-60 minutes each session. It represents a full-body routine that works everything and is a good way to start your bodybuilding and life-altering journey.

3 Days per Week	
Squats	3-4 x 15-20
Bench Press	3-4 x 8-12
Bent-Over Row	3-4 x 8-12
Dips, Behind the Back	3-4 x 8-12
Curls	3-4 x 8-12
Hanging Leg Raises, Bent-Knee	2 x failure
Crunches	2 x failure

Bodybuilding: Full-Body Workout #5

Workout time: 30-45 minutes

This is a good introduction into the world of high-intensity, low-volume bodybuilding training. As indicated below, perform 1-2 working sets of each exercise for the prescribed number of reps (make sure you warm up with each exercise first—we don't count those warm-up sets). If you can't do 12 reps of the Chin-up exercises listed below, substitute any other type of chins (such as Inverted Pull-Ups) you can do for 12 reps. Take 2-3 minutes rest between sets.

3 Days per Week	
Crunches	1 x failure
Squats	2 x 20
Stiff-Legged Deadlifts	1 x 10
Chins (any type)	1 x 12
Bench Press	2 x 6
Bent-Over Row	2 x 8
Military Press, Seated	1 x 6
Curls	1 x 6
Calf Raises	1 x 15
Crunches	1 x failure

Bodybuilding: Full-Body Workout #6

Workout time: 30-45 minutes

This workout is straightforward and focus-driven—ten exercises, each for ten reps per set. Perform this low-volume, high-intensity workout three days per week (how about the venerable Monday, Wednesday, and Friday?). Make sure to do one or two light warm-up sets before each working set listed below. Other than the first exercise, you'll be performing two working sets of 10 reps for each exercise. After 6-8 weeks on this program, take a week of rest, then move up to a more advanced workout.

3 Days per Week	
Side Bends	1 x 10
Squats	2 x 10
Stiff-Legged Deadlifts	2 x 10
Calf Raises	2 x 10
Bench Press	2 x 10
Bent-Over Rows	2 x 10
Military Press, Standing	2 x 10
Curls	2 x 10
Extensions, Lying	2 x 10
Sit-Ups	2 x 10

Bodybuilding: Full-Body Workout #7

Workout time: 20-60 minutes

This workout introduces you to a few exercises you may have never performed before. The first two weeks, perform one set of 10-12 reps on each exercise. For weeks 3-6, perform two sets of 10 reps for each. For the abdominal exercises, try to work up to 15-20 reps. Take 1-2 minutes rest between sets.

3 Days per Week	
Incline Press	1-2 x 10-12
One-Arm Row	1-2 x 10-12
Bent-Over Rear Delt Rows	1-2 x 10-12
Dips, Behind the Back	1-2 x 10-12
Curls	1-2 x 10-12
Wide-Grip Upright Rows	1-2 x 10-12
Reverse Curls	1-2 x 10-12
Front Squats	1-2 x 10-12
Good Mornings	1-2 x 10-12
Calf Raises, One-Leg	1-2 x 10-12
Hanging Leg Raises, Bent-Knee	1-2 x 15-20
Sit-Ups	1-2 x 15-20

Bodybuilding: Full-Body Workout #8

Workout time: 30-45 minutes

This classic higher-rep workout starts by warming you up with lots of core exercises—then proceeds to one exercise for each major muscle group (make sure to warm-up on each of these subsequent exercises). Take 1-3 minutes rest between sets, as necessary.

3 Days per Week	
Sit-Ups	1 x 15-50
Side Bends	1 x 15-50
Alternating Leg Raises	1 x 15-50
Bench Press	2-3 x 10-15
Military Press, Standing	2-3 x 10-15
Chins (any type)	2-3 x 10-15
Extensions, Standing	2-3 x 10-15
Curls	2-3 x 10-15
Squats	2-3 x 10-15

Bodybuilding: Full-Body Workout #9

Workout time: 30-45 minutes

This is full-body, high-intensity bodybuilding personified—you only get one shot at each exercise, so make it count. Unless otherwise directed, perform one set of each exercise for the prescribed number of reps (make sure you warm up with each exercise first—we don't count those warm-up sets). If you can't do 12 reps of the Chin-up exercises listed below, substitute any other type of chins you can do for 12 reps.

3 Days per Week	
Squats	2 x 20
One-Leg Calf Raises	2 x 20 (each leg)
Press Behind the Neck	1 x 12
Chins Behind the Neck	1 x 12
Bench Press	1 x 12
Bent-Over Rows	1 x 12
Dips, Behind the Back	1 x 12
Curls	1 x 12
Extensions, Standing	1 x 12
Chins to the Front	1 x 12
Dips, Behind the Back	1 x 12
Stiff-Legged Deadlifts	1 x 15
Wrist Curls, Behind the Back	1 x 12
Crunches	1 x 12

Bodybuilding: Full-Body Workout #10

Workout time: 30-60 minutes

This is a good workout to gauge how well your body handles and recovers from high volumes of work. Ten sets of each exercise with reps starting at ten and decreasing by one each set (10,9,8,7,6,5,4,3,2,1). Rest between sets should start at about one minute and decrease as the reps decrease—take more or less as you need it. Good luck.

3 Days per Week	
Front Squats	10 x 10,9,8,7,6,5,4,3,2,1
Bench Press	10 x 10,9,8,7,6,5,4,3,2,1
Pull-Ups	10 x 10,9,8,7,6,5,4,3,2,1
Deadlifts	10 x 10,9,8,7,6,5,4,3,2,1
Crunches or Leg Raises	2 x 15

Bodybuilding: Full-Body 4-Month Program

Workout time: 45-60 minutes

If you are a beginning weight trainer and serious about packing some serious muscle on your frame, then this full body routine will get you where you want to go. You'll need to work out three days per week, for 45-60 minutes each session. The suggested workout days are Monday, Wednesday, and Friday, although you can change that to anything that fits your schedule—just try to keep one rest day between each workout. This is a four month program—just follow the workouts below for the weeks indicated. As you progress, the volume of work and exercise variety increases, building a solid foundation of movement, strength, muscle and overall conditioning. For the first few weeks, take two minutes rest between sets, eventually decreasing the rest interval to a steady one minute. After completing the four months, you'll be transformed, amazed and amazing.

Weeks 1-2

3 Days per Week	
Hanging Leg Raises, Bent-Knee	2 x 10
Sit-Ups	2 x 10
Squats	2 x 8-10
Stiff-Legged Deadlifts	2 x 8-10
Calf Raises	2 x 8-10
Bench Press	2 x 8-10
Inverted Pull-Ups	2 x 8-10
Bent-Over Rows	2 x 8-10
Military Press, Standing	2 x 8-10
Wide-Grip Upright Rows	2 x 8-10
Curls	2 x 8-10
Extensions, Lying	2 x 8-10

Weeks 3-6

3 Days per Week	
Sit-Ups	2 x 15
Squats	3 x 8-12
Stiff-Legged Deadlift	2 x 8-12
Bent-Over Rows	2 x 8-12
Upright Rows	2 x 8-12
Dips, Behind the Back	2 x 8-12
Wrist Curls, Behind the Back	2 x 10-15
Calf Raises	3 x 10-15

Weeks 7-10

3 Days per Week	
Hanging Leg Raises, Bent-Knee	3 x 20
Squats	4 x 10-15
Stiff-Legged Deadlifts	3 x 8-12
Deadlifts	2 x 6-10
Inverted Pull-Ups	4 x 8-12
Shrugs	2 x 10-15
Military Press, Standing	3 x 6-10
Curls	3 x 8-12
Extensions, Lying	3 x 8-12
Wrist Curls, Behind the Back	2 x 10-15
Reverse Curls	2 x 10-15
Seated Calf Raises	4 x 10-15

Weeks 11-16

3 Days per Week	
Sit-Ups	2 x 20
Hanging Leg Raises, Straight Leg	2 x 15
Squats	4 x 10-15
Leg Curls	3 x 8-12
Deadlifts	3 x 6-10
Bent-Over Rows	3 x 8-12
Chins (any type)	2 x 8-12
Upright Rows	3 x 8-12
Military Press, Standing	3 x 6-10
Wide-Grip Upright Rows	2 x 8-12
Curls	3 x 8-12
Extensions, Lying	3 x 8-12
Reverse Curls	2 x 8-12
Wrist Curls, Behind the Back	3 x 10-15
Calf Raises	5 x 15-20

Bodybuilding: Full Body to Split-Body Transition Program

This routine takes the beginning weight trainer through a four week bodybuilding program, starting gradually with an introduction to full-body training, slowly increasing the workout volume, intensity and variety, culminating with a graduation to advanced split-body training by the fifth week.

Week 1

Workout time: 20 minutes, 3 days per week

Take two minutes rest between each set.

3 Days per Week	
Crunches	1 x 12
Hanging Leg Raises, Bent-Knee, One-Leg	1 x 12
Incline Press	1 x 12
Inverted Pull-Ups	1 x 12
Bent-Over Rows	1 x 12
Dips, Behind the Back	1 x 12
Curls	1 x 12
Squats	1 x 15
Stiff-Legged Deadlifts	1 x 15

Weeks 2–4

Workout time: 20-45 minutes, 3 days per week

For these next three weeks, you'll reduce the rest periods to one minute between each set, and perform one additional set of each exercise each week, until you are completing four sets of each exercise by week four.

3 Days per Week	
Hanging Leg Raises, Bent-Knee	2-4 x 12
Sit-Ups	2-4 x 12
Bench Press	2-4 x 12, 10, 10, 8
Bent-Over Rows	2-4 x 8-10
Curls	2-4 x 8-10
Dips, Behind the Back	2-4 x 10-12
Squats	2-4 x 15
Calf Raises	2-4 x 15-20

Weeks 5+

Workout time: 30-60 minutes, 3 days per week

Starting with week five, you'll migrate from the full-body workout scheme of the past four weeks to a more advanced split-body routine—working your upper body in **Workout A** and the lower body in **Workout B**. Keep alternating between these workouts, three days per week, until you feel ready to move onto one of the dedicated split-body routines. After completing this program, you'll be conditioned to volume, intensity, variety, success and failure—graduating Weight Training 101.

Workout A (Upper Body)		Workout B (Lower Body)	
Bench Press	3-4 x 12, 10, 8	Squats	4 x 12, 10, 8, 6
Chins (any type)	3-4 x 10-12	Stiff-Legged Deadlifts	3 x 10
One-Arm Row	3-4 x 8-10	Leg Curls	3-4 x 10-12
Military Press, Seated	3 x 8-10	Calf Raises	4 x failure
Wide-Grip Upright Rows	3 x 8-10	Seated Calf Raises	4 x failure
Curls	3-4 x 8-10		
Close-Grip Bench Press	3-4 x 12		

Split Body Workouts

Once you gain experience or decide to dedicate additional time to work specific areas of your body within a single workout, the natural progression is to move from total body workouts to split body workouts. These workouts do exactly what they say—they divide the physique into several components, training those parts on specific days.

This section presents workouts that divide the body into 2-5 components, requiring you to train 2-6 days per week, based on the specific split routine and your available time. Remember, these represent just a few of the millions of combinations of splits and exercise groupings you can arrange. Eventually, you'll find which combinations produce the greatest results for you.

Let's categorize the workouts by how many parts the body is divided into.

2-Way Splits

2 Days per Week		
Workout #1	Workout A	Legs, Chest, Upper Back, Abs
	Workout B	Lower Back, Shoulders, Arms, Abs
Workout #2	Workout A	Hamstrings, Shoulders, Back, Triceps, Abs
	Workout B	Thighs, Calves, Chest, Traps, Shoulders, Biceps, Abs
Workout #3	Workout A	Chest, Back, Abs
	Workout B	Legs, Arms, Abs

3 Days per Week		
Workout #4	Workout A	Shoulders, Traps, Arms
	Workout B	Back, Chest, Legs

3-5 Days per Week		
Workout #5	Workout A	Shoulders, Back, Chest, Traps, Arms
	Workout B	Thighs, Hamstrings, Calves, Abs

4 Days per Week

Workout #6	Workout A	Chest, Shoulders, Arms, Calves
	Workout B	Back, Legs, Abs

6 Days per Week

Workout #7	Workout A	Abs, Chest, Shoulders, Back
	Workout B	Abs, Legs, Arms

3-Way Splits

3 Days per Week

Workout #8	Workout A	Legs, Back
	Workout B	Abs, Calves, Arms
	Workout C	Chest, Shoulders

3 Days per Week

Workout #9	Workout A	Lower Back, Chest, Abs
	Workout B	Upper Back, Biceps, Calves, Abs
	Workout C	Legs, Shoulders, Triceps

6 Days per Week

Workout #10	Workout A	Abs, Chest, Shoulders, Triceps
	Workout B	Abs, Upper Back, Biceps, Calves
	Workout C	Abs, Legs, Lower Back

4-Way Splits

4 Days per Week		
Workout #11	Workout A	Chest, Shoulders
	Workout B	Thighs, Calves, Abs
	Workout C	Back, Traps, Hamstrings
	Workout D	Arms, Abs

5-Way Splits

5 Days per Week		
Workout #12	Workout A	Back, Abs
	Workout B	Chest
	Workout C	Legs, Abs
	Workout D	Shoulders, Traps
	Workout E	Arms, Calves, Abs

If you have ample time and desire, training six times per week *may* accelerate your mass gains. However, more is not necessarily better. You'll need to gauge your recovery ability if you decide to embark on a six day per week regimen. (If you find it hard to go to sleep, lack the enthusiasm to train or become irritable, those are sure symptoms of over-training—you'll need to cut back.) With six training days, you have the option to split your body into two or three separate sessions, performing each workout three or two times per week, respectively.

Bodybuilding 2-Way Split: Workout #1

Workout time: 15-45 minutes

For this workout, perform 1-3 sets of each exercise for 6-10 reps on upper body movements, and 10-20 reps on lower body exercises. Take 1-2 minutes rest between sets. Suggested workout days are Monday and Thursday, although you can change that to anything that fits your schedule—just try to keep two rest days between each workout.

Monday

Target Area	Exercise	Sets	Reps
Legs	Squats	1-3	10-20
Chest	Bench Press	1-3	6-10
Low Back	Good Mornings	1-3	6-10
Calves	Calf Raises or Seated Calf Raises	1-3	10-20
Forearms	Wrist Curls, Behind the Back	1-3	6-10
Abdominals	Crunches	1-3	10-20

Thursday

Target Area	Exercise	Sets	Reps
Hamstrings	Sumo Deadlift or Stiff-Legged Deadlift	1-3	10-20
Shoulders	Military Press, Standing	1-3	6-10
	Wide-Grip Upright Rows	1-3	6-10
Biceps	Curls	1-3	6-10
Abdominals	Side Bends	1-3	10-20

Bodybuilding 2-Way Split: Workout #2

Workout time: 30-45 minutes

If you only have an hour or two per week to train, yet still have dreams of building bigger muscles, fear not—if you give everything you've got for 30-45 minutes twice per week, this routine will get you there. If you manage to find another 30 or so minutes in the week, do it three times per week. Always alternate between **Workout A** and **Workout B** each training session. Both workouts include some direct abdominal work for your core, although the deadlifts and squats will provide their own indirect effect on that area.

Workout A

Target Area	Exercise	Sets	Reps
Hamstrings	Stiff-Legged Deadlift	2	15, 10
Shoulders	Military Press, Standing	2	10, 6
Back	Pull-Ups	2	8-12
Triceps	Dips, Behind the Back	2	6-10
Calves	Calf Raises	2	25, 20
Abs	Hanging Leg Raises, Straight-Leg	1	10-20

Workout B

Target Area	Exercise	Sets	Reps
Thighs	Squats	2	15, 10
Chest	Bench Press	2	12, 8
Traps	Shrugs	2	15, 10
Shoulders	Military Press, Seated	1	8
Back	Chins (any type)	2	6-10
Biceps	Curls	2	10, 6
Calves	Seated Calf Raise	2	30, 25
Abs	Sit-Ups	1	15-20

Bodybuilding 2-Way Split: Workout #3

Workout time: 30-45 minutes

This workout is similar to the previous one but adds a lot more volume in the same time frame, so you'll need to really push yourself to get it completed in the recommended time. Because it's so similar to traditional strength training workouts (albeit with more volume and less rest), many categorize this type of workout a *Power Bodybuilding* routine. Alternate between **Workout A** and **Workout B** each time you train and give it everything you've got.

Workout A

Target Area	Exercise	Sets	Reps
Chest	Bench Press	4-5	15, 12, 10, 8, 6
Back	Chins (any type)	4-5	12, 10, 10, 10, 8
Chest	Incline Press	4-5	10, 8, 6, 6, 6
Back	Deadlifts	4-5	12, 10, 8, 6, 6
Abs	Crunches	2	15-20

Workout B

Target Area	Exercise	Sets	Reps
Thighs	Squats	5	15, 12, 12, 10, 8
Hamstrings	Stiff-Legged Deadlifts	5	12, 10, 8, 8, 8
Calves	Calf Raises	4	6-10
Biceps	Curls	4	6-10
Triceps	Dips, Behind the Back	4	10-12
Abs	Hanging Leg Raises, Bent-Knee	2	15-20

Bodybuilding 2-Way Split: Workout #4

Workout time: 10 minutes (beginner), 30 minutes (intermediate), 60 minutes (advanced)

The two workouts in this hypertrophy-based routine contain alternating pushing and pulling movements. Beginners should perform one set of each exercise, intermediates 1-3 sets, and advanced trainers can do 3-5 sets of each. Keep the reps in the 6-8 range for best results. Try this routine three days per week, alternating between each workout.

Workout A

Target Area	Exercise	Sets	Reps
Shoulders	Military Press, Standing	1-5	6-8
Traps	Shrugs	1-5	6-8
Triceps	Close-Grip Bench Press	1-5	6-8
Biceps	Curls	1-5	6-8
Abs	Sit-Ups or Crunches	1-5	12-15

Workout B

Target Area	Exercise	Sets	Reps
Back	Deadlifts	1-5	6-8
Chest	Bench Press	1-5	6-8
Back	Bent-Over Row	1-5	6-8
Thighs	Squats	1-5	6-8
Hamstrings	Stiff-Legged Deadlifts or Romanian Deadlifts	1-5	6-8
Calves	Calf Raises	1-5	6-8

Bodybuilding 2-Way Split: Workout #5

Workout time: 45-60 minutes

This training program is divided into upper and lower body workouts. You'll select one of the routines each workout, alternating between the two. You can perform this routine 3-5 days per week, based on your motivation, energy levels and recovery ability. For the first four weeks, perform two sets of each exercise—after that add an additional set and reduce your rest intervals from 2-3 minutes between sets to 1-2 minutes.

Workout A

Target Area	Exercise	Sets	Reps
Shoulders	Military Press, Seated	2-3	10-12
Back	Chins, To The Front	2-3	10-12
Chest	Incline Press	2-3	10-12
Shoulders	Bent-Over Rear Delt Row	2-3	10-12
Chest	Bench Press	2-3	10-12
Back	Bent-Over Row	2-3	10-12
Triceps	Dips, Behind the Back	2-3	10-12
Biceps	Curls	2-3	10-12
Shoulders	Wide-Grip Upright Rows	2-3	10-12
Forearms	Reverse Curls	2-3	10-12

Workout B

Target Area	Exercise	Sets	Reps
Hamstrings	Stiff-Legged Deadlift	2-3	12-15
Low Back	Good Mornings	2-3	12-15
Thighs	Front Squats	2-3	12-15
	Lunges	2-3	12-15
Calves	Calf Raises	2-3	12-15
Abs	Hanging Leg Raises, Bent-Knee	2-3	15-20
	Crunches	2-3	15-20

Bodybuilding 2-Way Split: Workout #6

Workout time: 45-60 minutes

In previous routines, you've seen how to split your body into two workouts and alternate between those each training day. Here it's the same protocol, except you'll double the frequency, performing each workout twice per week.

Monday & Thursday

Target Area	Exercise	Sets	Reps
Chest	Bench Press or Incline Press	5	6-12
Shoulders	Military Press, Standing or Seated	4	6-12
	Wide-Grip Upright Rows or Bent-Over Rear Delt Rows	3	8-12
Biceps	Curls	3	8-12
Triceps	Extensions, Seated	3	8-12
Forearms	Wrist Curls, Behind the Back	2	10-15
Calves	Seated Calf Raises	3	10-20

Tuesday & Friday

Target Area	Exercise	Sets	Reps
Back	Bent-Over Rows	4	6-12
	Chins (any type)	3	To failure
Thighs	Squats or Front Squats	5	6-12
	Lunges or Reverse Lunges	3	10-15
Hamstrings	Stiff-Legged Deadlifts	4	6-12
Calves	Calf Raises	3	10-20
Abs	Hanging Leg Raises (any type) or Crunches	3	15-20

Bodybuilding: 2-Way Split: Workout #7

Workout time: 45-60 minutes

With this routine you'll be training six days per week, alternating between two different workouts. Sunday is for rest. Amen.

Monday, Wednesday, Friday

Target Area	Exercise	Sets	Reps
Abs	Hanging Leg Raises (any type):	1	20
Chest	Bench Press or Incline Press	5	6-12
Shoulders	Military Press, Seated	4	6-12
	Wide-Grip Upright Rows	2	10-12
Back	Chins (any type)	3	To failure
	Bent-Over Rows	3	6-12

Tuesday, Thursday, Saturday

Target Area	Exercise	Sets	Reps
Abs	Crunches	1	20
Thighs	Squats or Front Squats	4	6-15
Hamstrings	Stiff-Legged Deadlifts	4	8-12
Low Back	Good Mornings	2	12-15
Biceps	Curls	2	8-12
Triceps	Extensions, Seated	2	8-12
Forearms	Wrist Curls, Behind the Back	2	10-15
Calves	Standing Calf Raises or Seated Calf Raises	3	10-15

Bodybuilding 3-Way Split: Workout #8

Workout Time: 15-30 minutes

For this workout, perform 1-3 sets of each exercise for 6-10 reps on upper body movements, and 10-20 reps on lower body exercises. Take 1-2 minutes rest between sets. Suggested workout days are (surprise!) Monday, Wednesday and Friday, although you can change that to anything that fits your schedule—just try to keep one rest day between each training session.

Monday

Target Area	Exercise	Sets	Reps
Thighs	Squats	1-3	10-20
Hamstrings	Stiff-Legged Deadlift	1-3	10-20
Back	Chins (any type) or Bent-Over Row	1-3	6-10

Wednesday

Target Area	Exercise	Sets	Reps
Abs	Crunches	1-3	10-20
	Side Bends	1-3	10-20
Calves	Standing Calf Raises or Seated Calf Raises	1-3	10-20
Biceps	Curls	1-3	6-10
Forearms	Wrist Curls	1-3	6-10
Shoulders	Wide-Grip Upright Rows	1-3	6-10

Friday

Target Area	Exercise	Sets	Reps
Chest	Bench Press	1-3	6-10
Shoulders	Military Press, Standing	1-3	6-10

Bodybuilding 3-Way Split: Workout #9

Workout time: 20-30 minutes

You aren't limited to dividing your bodybuilding program into two distinct workout sessions when training on a three day per week schedule. Here, we split the routine into three different workouts, each on their own day. This is a good power bodybuilding scheme if you can only devote about 30 minutes to each workout—now there are no excuses. Try it and watch how it packs on the muscle.

Monday

Target Area	Exercise	Sets	Reps
Back	Deadlifts	3	6
Chest	Incline Press	3	6
Abs	Weighted Crunches	3	12

Wednesday

Target Area	Exercise	Sets	Reps
Back	Chins (any type)	3	To failure
Biceps	Curls	2	6
Calves	Calf Raises	2	15
Abs	Crunches	1	To failure

Friday

Target Area	Exercise	Sets	Reps
Thighs, Hamstrings	Squats	3	8, 12, 12
Triceps	Dips, Behind the Back	2	To failure
Shoulders	Military Press, Seated	3	6
Calves	Seated Calf Raises	2	20

Bodybuilding 3-Way Split: Workout #10

Workout time: 45-60 minutes

Extending our last routine, here we add more frequency (now you are training six days per week), more volume within each workout, and increase the average rep range—therefore, you get a little more time to get through each workout.

Monday & Thursday

Target Area	Exercise	Sets	Reps
Abs	Hanging Leg Raises (any type)	1	20
Chest	Bench Press or Incline Press	5	6-12
Shoulders	Military Press, Seated	4	6-12
	Wide-Grip Upright Rows	2	8-12
Triceps	Extensions, Seated or Close-Grip Bench Press	3	6-12
Forearms	Reverse Wrist Curls	2	10-15

Tuesday & Friday

Target Area	Exercise	Sets	Reps
Abs	Crunches	1	20
Back	Chins (any type)	4	To failure
	Bent-Over Rows	4	8-12
Biceps	Curls	3	8-12
Forearms	Wrist Curls, Behind the Back	2	10-15
Calves	Calf Raises	3	10-20

Wednesday & Saturday

Target Area	Exercise	Sets	Reps
Abs	Hanging Leg Raises, Bent-Knee	1	20
Thighs	Squats or Front Squats	5	6-15
Hamstrings	Stiff-Legged Deadlifts	4	6-12
Lower Back	Good Mornings	3	10-15
Calves	Seated Calf Raises	3	10-20

Bodybuilding 4-Way Split: Workout #11

Workout time: 60 minutes

Over the past twenty years, I've had good success with this four-day per week routine, training each muscle group directly once per week. Because you only get one shot every week to train each muscle group, you tend to stay focused—the last thing you want to do is go easy and have to wait another week to redeem yourself. Each workout should take you about one hour.

A couple notes about this routine:

- Hamstrings are trained on a separate day from thighs, because most people tend to either neglect or not put enough effort into them.

- If you start with Bench Press one week, then start with the Incline Press the next week. Keep rotating in that fashion—it helps to develop the entire chest symmetrically.

- The Monday and Friday workouts are pushing and pulling days, whereas Tuesday is just pushing and Thursday is just pulling movements. Again, balance is harmony.

Monday

Target Area	Exercise	Sets	Reps
Chest	Bench Press	5	6-12
	Incline Press	5	6-12
Shoulders	Bent-Over Rear Delt Rows	3	8-12
	Military Press, Seated	5	6-12
	Wide-Grip Upright Rows	3	8-12

Tuesday

Target Area	Exercise	Sets	Reps
Thighs	Squats	5	6-12
	Front Squats or Hack Squats	5	6-12
Calves	Seated Calf Raises	4	8-20
	Standing Calf Raises	4	8-20
Abs	Hanging Leg Raises (any type):	3	15-20

Thursday

Target Area	Exercise	Sets	Reps
Back	Chins (any type)	5	To failure
	Bent-Over Rows	5	6-12
Traps	Shrugs	5	6-12
Hamstrings	Stiff-Legged Deadlifts	5	6-12

Friday

Target Area	Exercise	Sets	Reps
Biceps	Curls or Drag Curls	4	8-12
	Reverse Curls	4	8-12
Triceps	Close-Grip Bench Press	5	6-12
	Extensions, Seated	3	8-12
	Dips, Behind the Back	3	To failure
Abs	Crunches	3	15-20

Bodybuilding 5-Way Split: Workout #12

Workout time: 30-40 minutes

A lot of people like training Monday through Friday after work, taking the weekend off. If you're going to be a weekday warrior, do it right and train one muscle group on each day, for about 30-40 minutes (more for large muscle groups, less for smaller ones). Here's one example of how you might structure this type of routine.

For the inexperienced, there is a method to the (seeming) madness here. First, while your energy reserves are built up from a weekend of high-carb eating, you'll want to hit a large muscle group like the back. After that initial day of pulling movements, the next day you should push, so chest comes next on the menu. Legs are reserved for midweek and will drain most of your remaining energy (see, it really is *hump day*). Therefore, Thursday is relatively easy compared to the previous day's effort, and Friday is for arms, because every Friday is International Arms Day. Seriously, by Friday you'll be longing to get out of the gym and collapse into the weekend, so some smaller muscles like arms, calves and abs seems about right.

Monday

Target Area	Exercise	Sets	Reps
Back	Deadlifts	3	6
	Chins (any type)	3	To failure
	Bent-Over Rows	3	8-10
Abs	Crunches	2	To failure

Tuesday

Target Area	Exercise	Sets	Reps
Chest	Bench Press	4	6-8
	Incline Press	3	8-10
	Guillotine Press	3	12

Wednesday

Target Area	Exercise	Sets	Reps
Thighs	Squats or Front Squats	5	8-12
Hamstrings	Romanian Deadlifts or Stiff-Legged Deadlifts	4	8-12
Abs	Hanging Leg Raises (any type)	3	15-20

Thursday

Target Area	Exercise	Sets	Reps
Shoulders	Military Press, Standing or Seated	4	8-12
	Wide-Grip Upright Rows	3	10-12
	Bent-Over Rear Delt Rows	3	10-12
Traps	Shrugs	4	6-12

Friday

Target Area	Exercise	Sets	Reps
Biceps	Curls or Close-Grip Pull-Ups	4	8-12
	Reverse Curls	2	10-12
Triceps	Close-Grip Bench Press	4	6-10
Forearms	Wrist Curls, Behind the Back	2	12-15
Calves	Standing Calf Raises	3	12-15
	Seated Calf Raises	3	12-15
Abs	Hanging Leg Raises (any type)	2	15-20

SATURDAY & SUNDAY

God rested one day—here you get two.

Specialized Workouts by Muscle Group

Sometimes you just want to train hamstrings. Yeah, right.

Nine out of ten people that go to the gym, go there to specifically train one or two muscle groups. They pronounce, "Monday is chest and triceps", or "Tuesday is back day". (I'm not saying that's right or wrong—that's for you to determine.) If you are that person, this section is for you. Pick and choose from the workouts here to custom assemble your workout du jour.

Because we're talking hypertrophy-based bodybuilding training, where muscle size is our primary goal, each of the workouts below keep the reps in the time-tested 6-12 range for this purpose. Similarly, you'll see both classic higher-volume, moderate intensity workouts with anywhere from 8-16 sets per muscle group, to high-intensity, low volume workouts with only 4-8 working sets. Both are effective (remember—change is good).

Ultimately, after studying and completing each type of workout for all of the muscle groups below, you'll be able to modify and construct your own workouts, using the entire collection of exercises presented earlier.

Abs

High-Volume (10-15 min)		High-Intensity (3 min)	
Hanging Leg Raises (any type)	3 x 20	Weighted Sit-Ups	2 x 12
Crunches	3 x 20-25		

Back

High-Volume (30-45 min)		High-Intensity (20-25 min)	
Bent-Over Rows	4 x 6-8	Deadlifts	3 x 6
Chins, To the Front	3 x 10-12	Chins (any type)	3 x failure
One-Arm Rows	3 x 8-10	Bent-Over Rows	2 x 6-8
Chins, Behind the Neck	3 x 10-12		

Biceps

High-Volume (20-30 min)		High-Intensity (10 min)	
Curls	4 x 8-12	Close-Grip Pull-Ups (any type):	3 x failure
Reverse Curls	4 x 10-12		

Calves

High-Volume (25-30 min)		High-Intensity (10-15 min)	
Standing Calf Raises	5 x 10-20	Standing Calf Raises, One-Leg	2 x 15
Seated Calf Raises	5 x 10-20	Seated Calf Raises	2 x 15

Chest

High-Volume (25-40 min)		High-Intensity (15-20 min)	
Bench Press	5 x 8-12	Incline Press	3 x 6-8
Incline Press	5 x 8-12	Bench Press	3 x 6-8

Forearms

High-Volume (10-25 min)		High-Intensity (10 min)	
Wrist Curls, Behind the Back	4 x 10-15	Wrist Curls, Behind the Back	2 x 6-8
Reverse Wrist Curls	4 x 10-15	Reverse Wrist Curls	2 x 6-8

Glutes

High-Volume (25-40 min)		High-Intensity (10-15 min)	
Duck/Frog Squats	3 x 10-15	Duck/Frog Squats	2 x 8-12
Step Ups	3 x 10-15	Romanian Deadlifts	2 x 8-12
Romanian Deadlifts	3 x 10-15		
Reverse Lunges	3 x 10-15		

Hamstrings

High-Volume (15-25 min)		High-Intensity (10-15 min)	
Leg Curls	4 x 10-12	Romanian Deadlifts	4 x 6-8
Stiff-Legged Deadlifts	4 x 8-12		

Shoulders

High-Volume (25-40 min)		High-Intensity (15-20 min)	
Military Press, Seated or Press Behind the Neck	4 x 8-12	Military Press, Standing	3 x 6-8
Front Raise	3 x 10-12	Heavy Upright Rows	2 x 6-8
Wide-Grip Upright Rows	3 x 10-12	Bent-Over Rear Delt Rows	2 x 6-8
Bent-Over Rear Delt Rows	3 x 10-12		

Thighs

High-Volume (25-40 min)		High-Intensity (10-15 min)	
Squats	4 x 10-12	Squats	1 x 20
Front Squats	4 x 10-12	Front Squats	2 x 10-15
Lunges	4 x 12-15		

Traps

High-Volume (15-25 min)		High-Intensity (10-15 min)	
Shrugs	4 x 10-12	High Pulls	2 x 6
Upright Rows	4 x 10-12	Shrugs	2 x 6-8

Triceps

High-Volume (25-35 min)		High-Intensity (10-15 min)	
Close-Grip Bench Press	4 x 8-12	Close-Grip Bench Press	3 x 6
Extensions, Lying	4 x 10-12	Dips, Behind the Back	2 x failure
Dips, Behind the Back	3 x 10-12		

Other Approaches

A barbell and weight training in general, offers many life lessons. For example, there is a funny thing about weight training—the better you get at it and the longer you do it, the harder it becomes to improve. It's that damn law of diminishing returns. Eventually, everybody reaches a plateau. If you've progressed from full body to split-body workouts, perhaps even cycling back to full body workouts, with nary an ounce of new muscle growth in the past couple months, it may be time to try to other tactics. Sometimes, desperation provides the stimulus for change.

But first, take a week of complete rest. Often this will re-energize you both physically and mentally, remove you from any over-training miasma you may be trapped in, and prime your body for new growth and adaptation.

Here are some advance tactics you can use to increase strength and muscle mass.

One Exercise per Workout

Pick one exercise and do it for the entire workout. Sometimes in our hectic world this becomes a savior, a quest, and a day of satisfaction, all wrapped up in one single exercise, and unification of effort.

One Exercise with a Total Rep Target

Pick an exercise and some number of total reps you want to achieve and try to reach that number in as few sets as possible. Each time you do this, strive for that rep target using at least one less set to get there.

Chins are a good example. Let's say you decide you want to do 50 total reps. Starting chinning and continue until you can't perform another full rep. Take a break and do another set. Continue this process until you reach 50 reps. This rep-targeting technique works with any exercise and can be used across multiple exercises in a single workout session to provide a body-slam of muscle growth stimulus. Sometimes coaxing growth through progressive resistance stalls and you need to bring out the sledgehammer.

One Exercise per Muscle Group with Timed Sets

Pick a time limit for performing an exercise, let's say five minutes. Pick one exercise and perform it for as many reps as possible until you almost reach failure. Rest for 30 seconds and repeat the process until your five minutes are up. Of course, the five minute exercise block and 30 second rest intervals are variable—try shorter or longer time limits and rest intervals to determine their effect on your body. Record everything and strive to improve your performance next time. If you want to experience what maximum lactic acid build-up feels like, try this with calf raises.

◆ ◆ ◆ ◆

If none of these approaches work for you, it may be time for more drastic measures. Those are described in the **Intensity Techniques** section.

Combining Strength Training and Bodybuilding

Many strength purists disdain bodybuilding and the hypertrophy-focused, mirror-based umbrage it evokes, often stating they would rather be strong than just look strong. They have functional strength. Conversely, bodybuilders usually give a respectful nod to their strength training brethren, but choose to not be as strong if it requires drinking a gallon of milk a day and having a belly hanging over their belt. To both camps, I offer Tommy Kono, John McCallum and Fred Hatfield.

Olympic Weightlifting Gold and Mr. World

Tommy Kono won the gold medal in weightlifting at the 1952 and 1956 Olympic Games, as well as the Mr. World bodybuilding title in 1954. (Notice that the bodybuilding win was between Olympics, making it even more impressive.) Today, he's considered by many to be the greatest weightlifter of all time. So, it's really hard to argue with anything that comes out of his mouth. And Tommy embraced, talked about and wrote about combining both strength and bodybuilding-type training into a unified cyclical system. Typically, he would perform strength training exclusively for 6-8 weeks, and then switch to hypertrophy-style training for a few weeks to refresh his body and prepare for the next strength training onslaught. The same periodization approach can work for you.

If you want to try Tommy's approach, pick a workout routine from the strength training section, follow it for 6-8 weeks, then pick a workout routine from the bodybuilding section and try that for at least two weeks, then repeat the process.

The McCallum Approach

If you read to this point carefully, you'll remember I mentioned that John McCallum wrote *The Complete Keys to Progress*. He was also an advocate of dirt-simple, basic training built around low reps and heavy weights. His fictionalized stories (lessons) of friend Ollie and his daughter's boyfriend Marvin, eating cheese sandwiches and performing set after set of heavy dips, benches and squats are legend. That's strength training folks. But if you read through his stories, he has a further message—adding in some additional volume via higher rep sets of traditional bodybuilding-type movements (extensions, curls, calf raises) after the strength training work, produces a more muscular and strong physique. So, while Kono advocated an alternating cyclical approach to both types of training, McCallum combined them within every workout.

> **The typical McCallum approach for a basic exercise looks like this:**
>
> **3 sets of 5 reps, followed by 8 sets of 10 reps**

You'll notice that's a nice blend of the beginner's 3x5 method that Starr popularized and so many others, like Mark Rippetoe advocate, combined with the typical higher volume, higher rep bodybuilding approach. McCallum liked to use this methodology with presses, squats and dips. No surprise there.

If you want to try John McCallum's approach, pick an exercise for a particular muscle group and perform three sets of five reps, lower the weight and continue with eight more sets, at ten reps this time. No need to do any more work for that muscle group—it should be toast.

Fred Hatfield and Scientific Bodybuilding

Dr. Fred Hatfield is first and foremost a powerlifter—a world record powerlifter. In 1980, he set the world record in the squat in the 90kg (198 lbs.) weight class with a lift of 826lbs—a record that still stands today. He wasn't too shabby in other competitive lifts as well, benching over 500lbs and deadlifting over 700lbs in various competitions in the 1980s. As a powerlifter, Hatfield used periodization to improve his lifts. However, in 1984 Hatfield wrote *Bodybuilding: A Scientific Approach*, which detailed his research on combining strength training, bodybuilding-type training, and muscular endurance training into a single holistic regime.

This holistic approach to weight training centers on the science of muscle cells, where muscles are composed of distinct types of structures. In his book, Hatfield describes these components of a muscle cell, their relative sizes, and the best methods to overload each. All of these components occupy physical space—therefore contributing to the overall size of a muscle. This concept of constructing specific workouts in order to provide overload to each muscle cell component *within a single workout* represents the epitome of compressing the concept of periodization into a single training session. Behind all the science, holistic training is a just a fancy moniker for making sure you use an array of rep ranges in each workout in order to completely exhaust all the various types of muscles fibers, ensuring that all of them grow to maximum potential. It's Kono and McCallum codified.

With that background out of the way, here are the major muscle cell components, listed in order from largest to smallest, as a percentage of overall muscle cell size, and the most effective rep ranges and method of performance for overloading them:

Muscle Cell Component	% of Total Muscle Size	Appropriate Rep Range	Performance
Myofibrils	20-30%	6-12	High-speed, explosive performance
Sarcoplasm	20-30%	6-25	Normal speed
Mitochondria	15-25%	15-25 (60% 1RM)	Slow speed, with continuous tension
Capillaries	3-5%	15-25	Slow speed, with continuous tension
Connective tissue	2-3%	6-12	

Based on the components of each muscle cell, Hatfield's synthesized training revolves around a key concept, elicited by both Kono and McCallum:

Each muscle cell component responds best to a different form of stress—therefore every training session should include each method of overload for every muscle group trained.

To satisfy the science of muscle cell differentiation and adaptive stress, Hatfield's basic holistic training workout schema, which he called ABC Training, consisted of:

- Sets of 4-6 reps done explosively (muscular power)
- Sets of 10-15 reps done rhythmically (muscular size)
- Sets of 30+ reps done slowly (muscular endurance)

The 30 rep sets should take you at least one minute to complete—if it's any shorter, you're lifting too quickly. Aim for one to two minutes per set. Performed correctly, these are grueling affairs.

Typically, basic compound movements such as squats, rows, deadlifts and presses are executed explosively for lower reps, whereas isolation exercises (curls, pushdowns, laterals, extensions) are performed rhythmically for higher reps.

To get you started, here are some examples of muscle groups and associated exercises using this approach. Start with one set of each and work your way up to three sets.

Back

Exercise	Reps	Performance
Bent-Over Rows	5-8	Explosive
Chins (any type)	10-15	Rhythmically
One-Arm Rows	20+	Slowly

Biceps

Exercise	Reps	Performance
Curls	5-8	Explosive
Inverted Close-Grip Pull-Ups	10-15	Rhythmically
Drag Curls	20+	Slowly

Calves

Exercise	Reps	Performance
Seated Calf Raises	5-8	Explosive
Standing Calf Raises	10-15	Rhythmically
Squatting Calf Raises	20+	Slowly

Chest

Exercise	Reps	Performance
Bench Press	5-8	Explosive
Push-Ups	10-15	Rhythmically
Guillotine Press	20+	Slowly

Hamstrings

Exercise	Reps	Performance
Romanian Deadlift	5-8	Explosive
Leg Curls	10-15	Rhythmically
Straight-Leg Deadlifts	20+	Slowly

Quads

Exercise	Reps	Performance
Squats	5-8	Explosive
Jefferson Squats	10-15	Rhythmically
Sissy Squats	20+	Slowly

Shoulders

Exercise	Reps	Performance
Military Press, Standing	5-8	Explosive
Bent-Over Rear Delt Rows	10-15	Rhythmically
Wide-Grip Upright Rows	20+	Slowly

Traps

Exercise	Reps	Performance
High Pulls	5-8	Explosive
Upright Rows	10-15	Rhythmically
Seated Shrugs	20+	Slowly

Triceps

Exercise	Reps	Performance
Close-Grip Bench Press	5-8	Explosive
Extensions, Seated	10-15	Rhythmically
Extensions, Lying	20+	Slowly

Circuit Training

The real versatility of the Smith Machine (and weight training in general) becomes quite evident when you start performing circuit training style workouts. The same machine you can use to bench 300 pounds with can be used to squat and press 95 pounds for 20-30 reps in rapid succession. And the effect on your body is vastly different. The purpose of circuit training is to improve overall strength, muscle size and cardiovascular fitness while building a symmetrical physique. Because we're operating in the mid-point of that weight training continuum, you won't become the strongest, most muscular, or the king of cardio here, but you will become an overall well-conditioned individual.

One thing to note right away—make sure you have each exercise movement mastered before embarking for the land of high reps and little rest. More is not necessarily better especially if it's more incorrectly performed reps. Always favor the performance of fewer reps correctly than more reps poorly.

One of the intangible benefits of circuit training is that it provides a real sense of structured accomplishment when you complete an exercise, circuit, and finally, the workout. It helps to mentally decompose a seemingly long, arduous task into smaller, manageable pieces. People like that.

Circuit training on the Smith Machine should provide you with a quick workout that builds muscle and elevates your heart rate. At the core, circuit training is nothing more than a series of four or more exercises performed one after the other, with little to no rest between them.

Use this type of training on the Smith Machine when:

- The gym is crowed and you want to do a quick workout without waiting for equipment.
- You are short on time but big on enthusiasm and energy and want to get both weight training and cardio training done quickly.

You can perform circuit training workouts for your total body, upper or lower body, and your core midsection area. Additionally, you can also employ a Peripheral Heart Action (PHA), push/pull, push/push, or pull/pull strategy when moving from one exercise to the next.

Each of the workouts in this section is designed for you to load the Smith Machine once and use that same weight for all the exercises in the circuit. You may have to briefly lock the bar into position to get ready for the next exercise.

Let's take a look at each of your options.

PHA Circuit Training

The main concept of PHA circuit training is to force blood flow up and down the body by working every major muscle group while maintaining an elevated heart rate. This is accomplished by alternating upper body and lower body exercises—as muscles in the upper body are worked, the muscles in the lower body can rest, and vice-versa. The goal of PHA training is improved strength, muscle size, cardiovascular efficiency and flexibility.

Each PHA workout uses a series of sequences, where each sequence consists of a group of exercises to be performed non-stop for a prescribed number of reps. Each sequence is repeated two or more times, then the next sequence is started. Take rest between sequences only if necessary. Remember, work at a fast pace in order to maintain an elevated heart rate.

So, where do you want your heart rate to be?

PHA Target Heart Rate = (220-age) x 0.8

For example, if you are 30 years old, your heart rate should stay around 150 for most of your workout. You can use a simple wrist-based heart rate watch to monitor this number when you work out.

Here's a quick reference of other PHA Target Heart Rates by age:

Age	Target Heart Rate (beats per min)
20	160
25	155
30	150
35	148
40	144
45	140
50	136
55	132
60	128

Now, let's look at a typical PHA circuit training workout.

PHA Circuit Training Workout

Workout time: 15-20 minutes

Perform 8-10 reps on each exercise and cycle through each sequence 2-5 times. Take rest between sequences only if necessary.

Sequence 1 (15-20 reps)

1. Military Press, Standing
2. Crunches
3. Squats
4. Extensions, Standing

Sequence 2 (10-12 reps)

1. Chins (any type)
2. Good Mornings
3. Leg Curls
4. Curls

Sequence 3 (8-10 reps)

1. Floor Press
2. Side Bends
3. Overhead Squats
4. Dips, Behind the Back

Sequence 4 (12-15 reps)

1. Bent-Over Rows
2. Side Bends
3. Calf Raises
4. Shrugs

Full Body Circuit Training

These circuits will work your entire body, from your calf muscles all the way up to your neck, from front to back. It's up to you to stay focused and finish what you started.

10 Minutes

- Full Body Workout #4

10-15 Minutes

- Full Body Workout #1
- Full Body Workout #2
- Full Body Workout #3
- Full Body Workout #5
- Full Body —Workout #9

5-25 Minutes

- Full Body Workout #6

10-25 Minutes

- Full Body Workout #8

10-30 Minutes

- Full Body Workout #7

Circuit Training: Full Body Workout #1

Workout time: 10 minutes

This is a good introduction to full-body circuit training. It will provide you with your first insight and experience of just how different circuit weight training is from traditional strength or hypertrophy-based training, and the effects it has on your system. And it'll be over in ten minutes. Start light.

Perform 10 reps of each exercise, 3 circuits, with one minute rest between circuits.

1. Military Press, Standing
2. Romanian Deadlift
3. Bent-Over Rows
4. Squats
5. Lunges
6. Curls

Circuit Training: Full Body Workout #2

Workout time: 10-15 minutes

This time, you'll increase the volume of the workout via additional circuits, allowing yourself a little more time to recover between circuits, as well.

Perform 10 reps of each exercise, 3-5 circuits, with 1-2 minutes rest between circuits.

1. Squats
2. Push Press
3. Bent-Over Rows
4. Lunges
5. Hanging Leg Raises, Bent-Knee

Circuit Training: Full Body Workout #3

Workout time: 10-15 minutes

Here, the volume increases again, through an additional exercise within the circuit. Perform 10 reps of each exercise, 3-5 circuits, with 1-2 minutes rest between circuits.

1. Romanian Deadlift
2. Bent-Over Rows
3. Upright Rows
4. Front Squats
5. Push Press
6. Lunges

Circuit Training: Full Body Workout #4

Workout time: 10-15 minutes

Perform 10 reps of each exercise, 3-5 circuits, with 1-2 minutes rest between circuits.

1. Squats
2. Deadlifts
3. Push-Ups
4. Lunges
5. Pull-Ups
6. Military Press, Standing

Circuit Training: Full Body Workout #5

Workout time: 10-15 minutes

This workout uses 8 reps for each of the 8 exercises; therefore you could call it an 8x8 circuit. Note that the sixth and seventh exercises are combined into one continuous movement, where you perform a squat immediately followed by a standing press. Right there, that's a full-body exercise combination.

Perform 8 reps of each exercise, 3-5 circuits, with 1-2 minutes rest between circuits.

1. Bent-Over Rows
2. Upright Rows
3. Military Press, Standing
4. Good Mornings
5. Lunges
6. Squats + Push Press
7. Romanian Deadlift

Circuit Training: Full Body Workout #6

Workout time: 10-15 minutes

By now, you should be well conditioned to circuit training—therefore, let's reduce the rest interval between circuits back to just one minute.

Perform 8-10 reps of each exercise, 3-5 circuits, with one minute rest between circuits.

1. Military Press, Standing
2. Pull-Ups
3. Floor Press
4. Bent-Over Rows
5. Deadlifts
6. Squats
7. Crunches
8. Split Squats

Circuit Training: Full Body Workout #7

Workout time: 10-25 minutes

Up till now, you've been performing circuit training workouts that last 15 minutes, at most. Let's increase the workload again, by increasing the reps and number of circuits. Start with three minute rest periods between circuits and gradually reduce that to one minute as your body adapts to the workout.

Perform 10 reps of each exercise, 3-5 circuits, with 1-3 minutes rest between circuits.

1. Squats
2. Deadlifts
3. Lunges
4. Calf Raises
5. Floor Presses
6. Upright Rows
7. Shrugs

Circuit Training: Full Body Workout #8

Workout time: 10-25 minutes

This is the longest full body circuit in this section. If you can make it through five circuits in less than 15 minutes, your cardiovascular conditioning and muscular endurance will be exceptional. And you should look damn good.

Perform 10 reps of each exercise, 3-5 circuits, with 1-3 minutes rest between circuits.

1. Squats
2. Push-Ups
3. Lunges
4. Bent-Over Rows
5. Deadlifts
6. Upright Rows
7. Dips, Behind the Back
8. Calf Raises
9. Curls

Circuit Training: Full Body Workout #9

Workout time: 10-25 minutes

By now, you should be highly conditioned to circuit training, so let's ramp up the number of circuits to eight and see how you handle that volume. For this circuit, you'll use a flat exercise bench with the Smith Machine. Keep it stationed there throughout the circuit—you can straddle the bench to perform the Rack Pulls. You might notice this circuit pays homage to traditional powerlifting.

Perform 10 reps of each exercise, 3-8 circuits, with 1-3 minutes rest between circuits.

1. Bench Press
2. Bench Squats or Bench Front Squats
3. Partial Deadlifts ("Rack Pulls")

Split Body Circuit Training

Although traditional circuit training is commonly used to work the entire body in a single session, there are occasions when you are limited by time or want to inject some bodybuilding-style split body training into your routine. That's where upper and lower body, as well as core circuit training routines become useful. This also allows you to increase the frequency of your circuit training sessions, because you can rotate between upper body, lower body and core circuit training each day. Here are some sample workout templates for each type. As you gain experience with these types of workouts and weight training in general, you'll be able to modify and then originate your own.

Upper Body Push/Pull Circuit

Workout time: 15-20 minutes

This workout alternates pushing exercises (Push-Ups, Dips Behind the Back) with pulling exercises (Pull-Ups, Bent-Over Rows). Perform 10-15 reps per exercise, 3-5 circuits, with 1-2 minutes rest between circuits.

1. Push-Ups
2. Pull-Ups (any type)
3. Dips, Behind the Back
4. Bent-Over Rows

Lower Body Push/Pull Circuit

Workout time: 15-20 minutes

This workout uses the traditional push/pull methodology to structure the exercise order. Remember to select a weight that you can perform with each exercise without changing the weight throughout the circuit. This might mean you have to increase the reps for lower body pushing exercises (squats), so that you can move to other pulling (deadlifts) and pushing (calf raises) movements without stopping to reset the weight.

Perform 10 reps per exercise, 3 circuits, with 1-2 minutes rest between circuits.

1. Squats
2. Straight-Leg Deadlifts
3. Calf Raises
4. Jefferson Squats
5. Romanian Deadlifts
6. Squatting Calf Raises

Core Circuit—Workout #1

Workout time: 5-15 minutes

This circuit training workout is all about strengthening your core abdominal, oblique and lower back muscles. Proper exercise selections and ordering, focusing on standing movements that strengthen the core, are at the heart of this template design. Perform 8 reps per exercise, 3-5 circuits, with 1-2 minutes rest between circuits.

1. Overhead Squats
2. Squats
3. Good Mornings
4. Bent-Over Rows
5. Deadlifts

Core Circuit—Workout #2

Workout time: 10 minutes

This time we'll borrow the low-rep, heavier weight strength training scheme, combine it with the no-rest foundation of circuit training and select exercises which stress the core muscles of the midsection. Perform 5 reps per exercise, grind through 4 circuits, and rest only one minute between those circuits. After these ten minutes you'll know that you've had a productive workout.

1. Upright Rows
2. Overhead Squats
3. Good Mornings
4. Standing Press Behind the Neck
5. Bent-Over Rows

Circuit Training with Low-Back Issues

If you have chronic low-back issues that are manageable and you want to perform circuit training on the Smith Machine, it's advised that you minimize movements with compression to the spine. Basically, that means using an exercise bench for support where possible, using chins instead of rows for training back and employing the machine's safety mechanism to limit squat-depth range, if you are able to squat at all.

Here's an example workout you may want to try if the circuit training workouts listed previously are bothering your lower back. Try to keep the bench under the Smith Machine for as much of the workout as possible. For example, when moving from the Seated Military Press to Upright Rows, leave the bench as positioned and straddle it when performing the Upright Rows. Likewise, if you perform Inverted Pull-Ups for your chinning movement, lock the bar in a higher position and place your heels on the bench to perform the chins.

1. Military Press, Seated
2. Upright Rows
3. Chins (any type)
4. Bench Front Squats
5. Curls
6. Extensions, Lying
7. Bench Press

Cardiovascular Training

An interesting thing happened in 1996. Professor Izumi Tabata of Ritsumeikan University formalized his research results regarding high-intensity intermittent training. Much of this research was based on the training techniques he followed as a coach for the Japanese Olympic speed skating team, where the athletes would work in short bursts of maximum effort followed by very brief periods of rest. Specifically, twenty seconds of intense work were followed by ten seconds of rest, repeated continually for four minutes—what came to be called the Tabata Protocol. The results of Professor Tabata's research and further verification by other academic studies concluded that the Tabata Protocol produced similar effects on the body as steady state cardio exercises, but with additional anaerobic benefits as well (that's muscle-building stuff). That means you're working both the aerobic and anaerobic systems at the same time, similar to PHA circuit training. The real finding here is that after performing an exercise using the Tabata Protocol it's not uncommon for your resting metabolic rate to be elevated *for up to twenty four hours*. That burns serious calories.

Although Professor Tabata and other researchers verified the effectiveness of this protocol, the Soviets knew about it decades earlier. Damn Soviets.

Pair the Tabata Protocol with the Smith Machine and you've just turned your weight training device into an effective cardio workhorse. Using an appropriate Smith Machine exercise, you should be able to get about 65-70 reps in those four minutes (that's 8-9 reps per 20-second interval)—if you are even able to count at that point. It'll be the longest four minutes of your life. Think of it as High-Intensity Interval Training (HIIT), taken to the extreme. X-Games Cardio, anyone? Many world-class athletes now incorporate this type of training into their regimens—if they want to win. If you choose to incorporate this into your training, expect to lose some serious body fat while transforming your cardiovascular system.

Due to the extreme high-intensity of this method, Tabata-style training is recommended for advanced trainers only—even then, you may want to do this only once per week and gauge your body's response and recovery from there as to frequency.

The Tabata Protocol works best with multi-joint, compound movements like the squat, front squat, deadlift, and presses. The more muscles you can activate per rep, the greater the systemic effect. Because we're doing high-reps with little rest between sets, this will quickly accelerate your heart rate. Oh, and you're going to use relatively light weights with this. For guys out there, using just 65-95lbs on Tabata Front Squats is impressive. Try it.

As a final note, always make sure you warm-up properly before starting a Tabata session.

Let's sum this up.

The Tabata Protocol

- **20 seconds of exercise**
- **10 seconds of rest**
- **Repeat for 4 minutes**
- **Lie on ground for a while**

Beyond using Front Squats with the Tabata Protocol, here are some of the other Smith Machine exercises you may want to try with it as well:

- Deadlifts
- Sumo Deadlifts
- Squats
- Overhead Squats
- Zercher Squats
- Standing Military Presses

Weak Point Training

We all have them—weak and lagging muscle groups; problem areas. Most women obsess about them and men tend to ignore them. This is perhaps the hardest part of successful weight training, the most arduous part of the journey toward reaching your ultimate goal. The identification, acknowledgement, planning, and execution to eliminate these weak areas require intelligence, honesty, commitment and perseverance. It's the key to continuous progress in just about any endeavor.

Here, we can use the Smith Machine's inherent strengths of balance and stability, muscle isolation, and constant tension for corrective action. Often, weaknesses generate from failure to execute proper form throughout the entire range of motion. For many exercises, corrective form can be reinforced using the Smith Machine's rail-driven system. Because there are no motor path deviations possible here, you learn to pull that Bent-Over Row right into the appropriate part of your torso, and learn to feel those hamstrings fully stretch and contract on Stiff-Legged Deadlifts without fear of losing your balance. You can squat to complete failure without spotters.

The purpose of weak point training is to improve those lagging muscle groups, provide proportional strength and development, eliminate those problem areas and provide you with peace of mind, satisfaction and safety. Think of it as future-proofing your body. It will require some alteration of your existing workout regime. In fact, you may need to deliberately imbalance your current routine temporarily, via increased priority and workload for the weak area, in order to bring balance back to your physique. Failure to acknowledge or dismissal of these weak areas will lead to either an eventual halt in your physical progress or injury—likely both.

Are you willing to correct these problems? That's the first step.

Keys to Improving Weak Points

- Evaluation, identification and acknowledgement of weaknesses

- Verify that you are using correct form at all times

- Train weaknesses frequently—increase the workload volume

The last point bears some further explanation. How can we train something more frequently in conjunction with our existing workout schedule/regime? There are a couple ways to do this:

- Priority—train weaknesses first in the workout

- Frequency—inject sets for the weak area into your regular workout

- Exclusivity—train the weak area exclusively on its own day

The remainder of this section will identify common physique weaknesses in both men and women, and provide you with some ideas of how to plan and execute their elimination.

Optimal Physique Structures for Men & Women

The ancient Greeks had it right. Zeus, Apollo, Ares, Hercules, Perseus and the other mythological Greek gods, half-gods and heroes all shared the physical embodiment of the ideal man—wide shoulders, narrow waists, and large calves with strong, thick torsos and muscular legs. This ancient Greek male ideal forms the basis of muscular strength, power, size and aesthetics for the modern X-frame. This is what you should be aiming for—that structure will serve you well, regardless of your ultimate weight training goal.

This X-frame works for women too. The Greeks portrayed Athena, Artemis, and Hera as strong-willed women with a balance of strength and feminine aesthetics through an hour-glass form of narrow waists, tight arms, and shapely legs and derrières. This ideal is evident in the current crop of female fitness models and natural bodybuilders—and not the weakly inspired girls of the beauty pageants or the unseemly excess of chemical-laden female bodybuilders. Female legs do contain hamstrings. Sir Mix-a-Lot sang to us that glutes are glorious (and powerful). And it's ok to shed the shoulder pads of the 1980s and build a little of your own. Muscle accentuates the beautiful lines of the female body. Fat hides it.

Keep these images in your mind as you work to eliminate your weak points and build to your strengths.

Typical Weaknesses/Problem Areas for Men & Women

Although each of us is unique from a genetic perspective, it's surprising how similar the problem areas are for men and women as a collective. Most of that is due to lack of training balance. Let's take the men first. A lot of men exhibit small upper chest musculature, triceps the same size or smaller than the biceps, a narrow back, and overall lack of leg mass. For women, the clarion cry is familiar—flabby back of the upper arms and lack of leg shape, especially the hamstrings and calves. We can fix this.

Abdominals

Weak Upper Abs

Typically, this isn't a problem, because most of use learned how to do sit-ups as children in school. However, if you find your upper abs weak or underdeveloped, perform **Sit-Ups**, **Weighted Sit-Ups**, and **Crunches** in your workout.

Weak Lower Abs

This is especially common, and in fact, is one of the culprits in lower back problems. The root cause here is due to specificity. For most of your life, you've been bending over at the waist to pick things up. However, how often in your daily routine do you move your pelvis up towards your chest? Almost never—unless you are a gymnast or work for Cirque de Soleil. The fix is to perform reverse crunch exercises, such as **Hanging Reverse Crunches**, on a consistent basis.

Back

In general, back weaknesses are often caused by the relative imbalance between a person's pushing capability versus their pulling and hinge capabilities. Guys love to bench press, but don't spend similar amounts of time or effort with pulling movements, such as chins, deadlifts and rows. Often, the fix here is simply to balance the amount of work you perform for both your pushing and pulling movements. Remember, the body operates as a single unit, so keeping everything in balance tends to sort things out.

Lower Back

Deadlifts and **Good Mornings** are what you want here. Don't neglect the Good Mornings—they are both an excellent exercise to teach and learn the hip hinge, as well as a direct hit on the spinal erectors of your lower back.

Upper Back

Use a wide-grip on **Bent-Over Rows**. Also, **One-Arm Rows** are useful as well if you pull your hand to the middle of your rib cage and hold that contraction for a second or two. Those sore little muscles you feel the next day in your upper back are your rhomboids. Develop those and watch your posture improve.

Middle Back Thickness

Again, you want to use a wide-grip on **Bent-Over Rows** here. Make sure you hold each rep at the top for a tight squeeze.

Back Width

The wider your grip on **Chins** (any type), the more effect it will have on your back width—to a certain extent. Try using a grip slightly wider than shoulder width and gradually expand to wider grips, one finger at a time, until you get the effect you desire. Also, don't make the common mistake of performing partial reps with Chins. Start from a dead hang and pull until your chest touches the bar or your chin clears the bar. As noted strength coach Dan John would say, that's "the correct way".

Outer Back

Here, we're not talking about back width, but the level of development (thickness) in the outer back. So, thinking logically, if we used a wide-grip to target the middle back, shouldn't we use a narrow grip to target the outer back? Yes, we should. **Narrow-grip Bent-Over Rows** it is.

Biceps

For most guys, this area isn't a problem because, well, after chest you work biceps then go home, right? No problem with specificity, volume and consistency there. Just be aware that biceps are relatively small muscles compared to thighs, chest and back, so take that into consideration for volume, frequency and rest. To the ladies I say, don't just settle for shapely legs when you can have the same for arms as well, so start here.

Mass

Everybody seems to forget this, but before barbells were invented, man was able to develop large biceps by pulling himself up tree limbs and rock ledges using a close-grip. Take a look at modern male gymnasts. They perform a little exercise called the rings, which not only requires them to pull themselves up, but hold themselves in that position for an extended period of time. So, channel Bart Conner and make the **Close-Grip Pull-Ups** or **Inverted Close-Grip Pull-Ups** a staple in your routine. Both the **Curls** and **Drag Curls** should help you here too.

Outer Thickness

The same logic as the grip-width on rows for your back applies here as well. **Curls with a close-grip** affect the outer biceps thickness.

Inner Thickness

By now you know the grip-width drill. **Curls with a wide-grip** affect the inner biceps thickness.

Calves

Although genetics plays a large role in your overall calf development potential, consistent use of linear progression using impeccable form and full range of motion will go a long way toward maximizing that potential. Treat calf work as first-class citizens and they will respond.

Range of motion is essential with calf training—maybe more so than with any other muscle group. Think about it this way. When you walk, you work your calves, but only through a partial range of motion. Your calves do not start each step in a fully stretched position and they don't end in a fully contracted position. You're working that middle range of motion for most of your life. Make the calves work through those other two extremes (full stretch and full contraction), and that's where they really start to grow. Because range of motion is so critical to direct calf work, **Donkey Calf Raises** excel here, due to the pre-stretch that occurs with every rep.

One other point—heavy people don't have small calves. Getting stronger on squats and deadlifts by handling heavier weights will grow your calves. They have no choice if they want to hold you upright and help propel you forward.

If you need improvement in this area, train your calves often, work them in isolation (one-leg varieties), use heavy weights and both high and low-rep schemes, and make them a priority.

Upper Calves

It's rare that an individual would have weak upper calves and good lower calves, but if you find yourself in this situation, alter how you perform **Calf Raises** by holding each rep for 2-3 seconds in the fully contracted position. Also, try partial reps using only the top half of the movement—you should be able to increase the weight you use with this technique.

Lower Calves

As discussed earlier, your calves are comprised of two main muscles—the gastrocnemius and the soleus. The soleus gives the calves that aesthetic diamond shape when the legs are viewed from the front. They also attach below the back of the knee and low on the tibia. This is the key to understanding how to improve them. Because the seated calf raise positions your legs bent at the knee, they place proportionately more stress on the soleus (since the gastrocnemius is slack). Modify your workout to include more **seated calf raise** work versus either standing or donkey calf raises. Additionally, try performing seated calf raises using only the lower half of the movement. Finally, when performing standing calf raises, execute them with your legs slightly bent—this will shift more stress onto the soleus.

Chest

Chest development suffers when you let your ego pick the weight or dictate your form. I'm talking to you, guys. The ladies don't seem to have this issue of insecurity, maybe because there aren't that many ladies bench pressing. That's too bad, because the bench press is an equal opportunity developer.

Upper Chest

I've never observed anyone with an overly developed upper chest, one that was imbalanced with the lower chest. I'm placing bets right now that I never will. One of the primary reasons why upper chest development lags behind is simply gravity and fortitude. Pressing a weight directly overhead is one of the toughest things to do in weight training. Pressing a heavy weight overhead when lying at an inclined angle is just slightly less foreboding. To fix this imbalance, which is especially important for the aesthetics of bodybuilding, as well as a great assistance lift for powerlifters, you need to—yes, do more incline pressing. To bring this area into relative balance, I recommend starting with incline presses two out of every three chest workouts, until things improve noticeably, then switch to an every other workout strategy. Additionally, don't forget the value of **Guillotine Presses** here. Finally, experiment with the angle of the bench—some individuals respond to lower angles in the 20-30 degree range, whereas others respond best to higher angles (40-45 degrees). Let your structure dictate your angle.

Lower Chest

Although you might never witness someone with overly developed upper pectorals, you also usually don't see much direct work for the lower chest being necessary. The standard bench press should effectively build this area. However, if you think you need more work here, use **Decline Presses** obviously.

Outer & Inner Chest

Problems with lack of outer and inner chest development are easily addressed through grip-width changes and are another reason to occasionally modify your grip through a planned periodization scheme. Here, performing flat, incline, or decline presses with a wider than normal grip will produce more affect to the outer regions, whereas closer grips will naturally target the inner area. Additionally, for inner chest problems, be sure to hold all pressing contractions for 2-3 seconds at the top of the movement. In fact, as you've probably noticed by now, that's a good general rule when addressing weaknesses. To place additional stress on the outer chest, try partial reps pressing the weight only halfway up.

Forearms

If you have weak or underdeveloped forearms, you probably aren't performing heavy deadlifts, rows, and shrugs. Most often, consistently holding onto a heavily loaded bar when performing those exercises (no straps, please) resolves this issue. If it doesn't, then you'll need to incorporate direct forearm work, which means wrist curls and reverse curls.

Inner Forearms

If you have forearm issues, usually this isn't the area. Why? Because bending your wrist toward you, which activates the forearm flexor muscles, is a common daily human movement. You do it when eating with utensils, picking things up, and shoveling. However, if you do need to improve this area, **Wrist Curls Behind the Back** targets these muscles and provides you with the best opportunity on the Smith Machine to get that full contraction.

Upper Forearms

This is where we usually see forearm imbalances. Why? Because bending your wrist *away* from you, which activates the forearm extensors, is not a common daily human movement. You see, your body and your lifestyle really do define you. To fix this imbalance, **Reverse Curls** and **Reverse Wrist Curls** will help. Remember to hold each movement at the top of each rep and squeeze the muscles for 2-3 seconds.

Glutes

The problem with glutes typically lies at the extremes—it's either too large or not there at all. If you have either issue, you know what I mean. If you think your butt is too big, your strategy is two-fold: reduce the amount of work that activates the glutes (less squats and deadlifts) and reduce your body fat level.

If you need to develop a rear end, first make sure you are incorporating enough direct work for that area—more squats, deadlifts, reverse lunges, etc. Second, verify that you are performing those exercises correctly. Although the squat is categorized primarily as a thigh exercise, it's really a complete lower-body builder, including thighs, hamstrings, glutes and calves. Remember, it's not about bending your knees, but rather dropping your torso straight down between your legs. Specific exercises that will really target the glutes include any wide-stance squats (**Duck/Frog Squats**), **Step Ups**, and **Lunges**, especially **Reverse Lunges**.

Hamstrings

Hamstrings are a lot like posterior (rear) delts—you just never see anyone with overly developed hamstrings. Often, it's just the opposite, especially with athletes. Weight trainers, runners, and other athletes realize they need to train their legs, but their legs often start and end with the thighs—and maybe some calf work if you play basketball or volleyball. Those hamstrings are important if you want to remain an injury-free participant in your chosen activity. How many times have you witnessed someone running, either on television or in person, suddenly pull up and grab the back of their leg? Typically, that's a pulled hamstring—or worse. Often, and apologies to Mr. Stallone, what just happened is they asked their body to write a check it couldn't cash. They have weak, underdeveloped hamstrings relative to their quadriceps. You see, it's not just an aesthetic thing here. The body likes, and often insists on a natural balance evolved over thousands of years. Here's how to correct this.

Mass

Squats and deadlifts (especially **Sumo Deadlifts**), performed correctly, will go a long way toward developing your hamstrings. Throw in some additional direct work, such as **Romanian Deadlifts** and **Stiff-Legged Deadlifts** to ensure they get the attention they deserve. If you discover you need to play some quick catch-up to your thighs, perform your hamstrings work first, before thighs, or train them on their own separate day. Also, remember that strong, muscular hamstrings are not built with leg curls.

Lack Shape

What leg curls are especially useful for are enhancing the overall shape of your hamstrings, if that is important to you. Think of them as concentration or preacher curls for your hamstrings. The scientific name for your hamstrings is *biceps femoris*. Notice the 'biceps' part of the name. That should be a big clue. To really maximize the results from leg curls, hold each rep in the fully contracted position for 2-3 seconds.

Thighs

If your thighs are weak or under-developed, ask yourself these questions: Are you squatting correctly? Are you squatting enough? Affirmative answers to both often negate any issues in the rest of this section. However, as a logic exercise, let's go through the typical problem areas with quadriceps.

Mass

There's just no way around this absolute truth. If you want strong, muscular thighs you must perform some type of squat movement. Traditional squats can't be surpassed for overall leg development—and by legs I mean quadriceps, hamstrings and calves. Most weight trainers struggle with squat depth. Full-range squats are the first barometer to achieving optimal leg development. A little further down that road, if you want to shift the primary emphasis to the thighs, front squats are your mana from heaven. The upright back position transfers the emphasis squarely to the quadriceps. If you want to gauge how strong your quads really are, full-range front squats will enlighten you. Remember, the Smith Machine safety mechanism provides you with confidence and a lack of excuses here.

Because most weight trainers typically perform partial range squats, led by ego, unfounded fears of knee injury, and a lack of inner fortitude, size in the upper portion of the thighs is often not a problem. Carrot-shaped thighs are. Half squats, where much heavier loads can be used than in full-range squatting, will provide the stimulus you need to strengthen and enlarge the upper thigh.

Lower Thighs

Lack of proportionate size in the lower thighs is a common problem. The culprit is almost always a lack of range of motion in all squatting movements. Get your thighs down to parallel or slightly below and watch the issue disappear.

For specific lower thigh training, perform squats, front squats, and hack squats using only the bottom half of the movement. This will keep continuous tension on the lower thigh and provide the stimulus you need to progress. Adjust the weights accordingly. You can also try squatting with your feet a little farther forward than normal. This is another area where the balance of the Smith Machine excels.

Outer Thighs (the "Sweep")

Now, here we are starting to get firmly into the aesthetic world of bodybuilding. Pure strength trainers don't really care about how much sweep their outer thighs have. To bodybuilders, it's one of the holy grails of lower body development. Don't understand what I'm talking about? Ok, picture this. If you look at your legs straight on in a full length mirror, notice the arc (or maybe lack thereof) where your thigh attaches into your knee, bows outward just like the bow of an archer, and finally, attaches into the hip area. What the Greeks were idealizing and what bodybuilders strive for, is a pronounced arc from knee attachment rising outward to mid-thigh, then arcing back into the hip. This is one of the major visual differences in women's legs between pure runway models (no outer shape to the thigh) and really fit women. So, how do you achieve this? Well, genetically your parents either gave it to you or not. Seriously, although genetics pre-determines a large portion of the ultimate development of this aesthetic, you can do some things to maximize your latent potential here.

Enter the **Front Squat** and **Hack Squat**, followed by their lesser kin, the squat with feet pointing straight and close together. Front squats are the movement that nobody wants to do, which means you need to do it. Nothing and I mean nothing will do more to march you down the path of outer thigh sweep domination than performing endless sets of front and hack squats. Why? Here science provides you with the answer. Thighs are quadriceps—"quad", meaning four pieces. Those two exercises place a disproportionate amount of stress on the *vastus lateralis*, the outer quadriceps muscle.

Inner Thighs

Strength athletes and powerlifters rarely have a weakness here. Why?—because they typically perform squatting movements with a wide stance (feet set wider than shoulder width) and toes pointing out at about 30degree angles. There's one of your answers.

For more direct work on the *vastus medialis* (the inner quadriceps muscle), perform **Stiff-Legged Deadlifts** and **Lunges**. Both of those exercises really help to fully stretch and contract that muscle area through a full range of motion.

Shoulders

Healthy, functional shoulders are all about balance. Imbalances are at the heart of most shoulder issues. Therefore, addressing problems here is about rebalancing. Because almost everyone performs far more pushing than pulling movements, it's typical for the posterior (rear) head of the deltoids to be relatively weaker and underdeveloped compared to the front of the shoulder, which absorbs much of the stress of pushing. Let's start there.

Rear of the Shoulder

To bring the rear shoulder into balance with the front, you need to perform as much pulling work as pushing. For most, that's a new adventure. Start your shoulder work with direct rear delt movements, such as **Bent-Over Rear Delt Pulls**. When performing **Bent-Over Rows** for your back, try bringing the bar up to your chest instead of the abdominal region, and holding it there for a second. You can also interleave a set of rear delt work with each of your regular workout sets. That's a good general strategy for correcting *any* weakness.

Front of the Shoulder

Due to the plethora of pushing exercises in a typical workout, lack of strength or development in the anterior (front) of the shoulder is rare. However, if you do require improvement here, **Military Presses**, **Incline Presses**, **Reverse Presses**, **Upright Rows**, and **Front Raises** will fix things quickly.

Shoulder Width

Again, the Greek ideal raises its head here. Both men and women want smaller waists. Nothing assists with the illusion of making your waist smaller than wider shoulders. Even if cursed by a relatively narrow scapula, the more muscle you can add to the lateral (side) head of your delts, the wider your shoulders become. What nature neglected you can grow. Conversely, if genetics blessed you with a wide shoulder structure, you can work to those strengths and accentuate the positive.

Typically, you target the side of your shoulders with dumbbell laterals. If all you've got is the Smith Machine, performing **Wide-Grip Upright Rows** emulates much of the benefit of that movement. Remember to hold the top position for a second or two and lower only about three-fourths of the way down. This provides a continuous time under tension effect on the lateral deltoids, increasing the effectiveness of the stimulus.

Traps & Neck

I've grouped these two together, because direct trapezius work typically takes care of any garden snake neck issues you may have. Although I haven't encountered many women who desire a bigger neck, failure to neglect one of the biggest parts of the back—the trapezius—creates more of those darn imbalances we should be concerned with.

Mass

Adding muscle mass to your traps and neck are not just about shrugging exercises. The trapezius is a kite-shaped, four-pronged muscle grouping which is involved with all pulling movements. The clue here should be obvious—heavy **deadlifts** (of all varieties) are the brute force Mack Truck™ movement for growing big, strong muscular backs—and backs include the trapezius. For more direct trap work, all varieties of **shrugs** and **upright rows**, as well as **Bent-Over Rows** with a wide grip and a 2-3 second contraction at the top will round things out.

Triceps

Now we arrive at one of the notorious problem areas for both women and men. Because women are from Venus and men from Mars, naturally both camps think their issues here are different when in reality they share the same villain—the long head of the triceps. Let's back up a little. Latin tells us that "tri" means three, so the triceps must be composed of three distinct muscles. And it is. The one we are concerned with here, the troublesome one of the bunch, is the long head, which runs all the way from the elbow up to the back of the shoulder. It's not only long, but big which is why most women complain of hanging, swinging backs of their arms, and why most guys complain about lack of arm size in general.

Dips and presses are the heart and soul of overall triceps development. Those simple movements will place stress across the entire triceps complex. However, to target that long head, you need to place that muscle in a position which elicits the greatest potential for stress possible, from full stretch to full contraction. Due to the attachment position of the long head, from elbow to rear shoulder, you need to perform extension movements that position your elbows pointing toward the top of your head throughout the exercise. For us on the Smith Machine, standing or seated extensions meet this requirement.

◆ ◆ ◆ ◆

Extra: Women's Six-Week Leg & Butt Specialization Program

Because so many women lament about the hideous nature of their legs, I've thrown in this extra special weak point training workout to help assuage these concerns. This is a specialized training program for women (but men can do it too!) that helps to build and shape the entire lower body. Additionally, it also firms the shoulders, arms and stomach, providing a knockout appearance that no one can miss.

Perform this routine three days per week, as indicated, for six weeks—alternating between **Workout A** and **Workout B** below. Typically, workout days are Monday, Wednesday, and Friday. Each workout should take you no longer than 45 minutes.

Workout A		Workout B	
Front Squats	5 x 15, 12, 10, 10, 10	Duck/Frog Squats	5 x 10
Stiff-Legged Deadlift	3 x 12	Lunges	3 x 10
Leg Curls	3 x 12	Leg Curls	3 x 10
Calf Raises	3 x 20	Lunges	3 x 10
Incline Press	4 x 10	Bent-Over Rows	3 x 12
Inverted Close-Grip Pull-Ups	4 x 10	Military Press, Seated	3 x 12
Crunches	4 x 25	Curls	3 x 12
		Dips, Behind the Back	3 x 12
		Seated Calf Raises	3 x failure
		Hanging Knee Raises, Bent-Knee	3 x 15

Injury Rehab & Prevention

Eventually, you will get injured during weight training. As you age, the specter of injury raises its head more often. Or, your injury might be the result of chronic overuse (the archenemy of consistency), or a slight hyperextension of a joint or overstretching a tendon. Like most other rewarding endeavors in life, with reward comes risk and intense weight training is an inherently risky activity. But, there are steps you can take to minimize and mitigate this risk. Additionally, when you find yourself in an injured state, there are proven and effective strategies for recovering from those injuries so that you can emerge better than ever. This section will show you how to both minimize and recover from injuries.

General Principles for Rehab & Recovery

By now, everyone knows the RICE principle—rest, ice, compression, elevation. If not, go look it up online. It usually works, and if not, can't make things worse.

In the early 1970s, with the publication of *Only the Strongest Shall Survive: Strength Training for Football*, Bill Starr outlined his ten principles for rehabilitating injuries. Those principles are applicable to any sport, and are particularly apt for anyone working through a weight-training injury, so I want to focus, and then expand the discussion around them.

1. Don't diagnose an injury.

Unless you're both a doctor and a weightlifter, don't try to play one in the gym or at home. As a first step after getting injured, go see your doctor for his or her diagnosis.

2. Refer all injuries to your doctor for diagnosis.

This one goes hand in hand with #1, above. I'll add one more detail to this.

Usually, your doctor is a general practitioner. *General* is the key word here. If the doc thinks you have anything seriously wrong, or that little voice in your head (the one you should always be listening to) says to ask for a more specialized opinion, then ask for a referral to another doctor. But not just any doctor. You want someone who is well respected in the area of your injury. How can you determine that? Find out who the specialists are that treat injuries for your local professional sports teams. If you live in an area that doesn't have any local pro sports teams, you should be able to find the sports medicine doctors that work with local universities and colleges. I suggest starting with the doctors associated with the pro teams first, because they deal with athletes that have millions of dollars invested in them and trust me they've been vetted and have proven their worth. Chances of them screwing up are minimal.

Here's a quick story to hammer this one home.

Many years ago, I had a training partner who lifted with me several days per week for over ten years (you tend to hold onto good training partners like *The One Ring* when you find them). After several years of training together, Jason starting having problems with his left shoulder. Because that type of injury is pretty common with long-time weightlifters, he tried rehabbing it on his own with a combination of anti-inflammatories, rest, ice, light weights, and higher reps. It didn't work, so he went to his family doctor. Because the shoulder only bothered him when he pressed heavy weights overhead, his doctor suggested that he stop doing that—forever. Onto the next doctor who basically said the same thing. Jason finally listened to his little voice and sought out the shoulder specialist for the Baltimore Ravens. She ordered an MRI, analyzed the results and told him he had a fully torn labrum. It required surgery if he wanted to resume his prior lifting. Jason had the surgery (which she performed), and after three months of carefully prescribed rehab, he was back to pressing heavy weights overhead with no problem. That was almost ten years ago and he's still going strong.

3. Don't exercise any injured area that results in acute pain.

Acute pain is a sudden, sharp pain. Dull pain is something else. You need to be able to recognize the difference. Have the courage to accept the answer and act accordingly.

4. Use very high reps for the first two weeks of rehab.

Using an exercise that works the injured area, Starr recommends starting with three sets of 25 reps every day for the first two weeks of rehab. You will probably be using a weight that's at least 50% less than your normal working weight. Don't try to do any other work for the injured area; otherwise you're just going to escalate the problem.

5. Work the injured area directly.

Although many practitioners advocate working around the injured area, Starr has you going right at it, using the high-rep approach described in #4, above.

6. Exercise the injured area every day during rehab.

This is especially important during the first two weeks of rehab. After that, you can gradually back off on the frequency and slowly lower the reps.

7. The injured area should receive exercise priority.

Work your injured area first in the workout. Don't wait until the end of the workout to perform those rehab sets. Your focus should be on recovering as efficiently and quickly as possible so act that way.

8. Progressively lower the reps and increase the weight.

After the first two 25-rep weeks, gradually increase the weight and lower the reps. As a first step, I recommend going from 25 reps to 20 reps. Additionally, start backing off on the frequency of work for the injured area. After the initial two weeks, switch from an everyday approach to an every other day system. As the weeks progress, move to 15 reps, then 12, and so on, always gauging your progress, performance, and recovery every step of the way.

9. Emphasize good nutrition during the recovery period.

Now is not the time to eat Pop-Tarts™, Lean Pockets™ or that crunchy taco supreme. Your body always thrives on natural, healthy foods, and never more so than when it's in an injured state. The body is trying to repair itself, to get back to homeostasis. Don't obstruct it. Drink lots of water. Eat foods that are as close to nature as possible ("If man made it, don't eat it." Thanks Jack.). You can never go wrong by eating lean proteins, fruits and vegetables. Healthy fats (nuts, olive oil) are especially good during these times.

10. Keep in contact with your doctor.

Not only common sense, but remember that your relationship with your doctor is about communication—and communication requires a two-way interaction. Your doctor appreciates feedback about how the rehab is progressing, and can make adjustments as necessary.

At this point, I'll add one more useful thing—partial reps.

Now, normally you want to be doing full-range reps, including during the rehab period. However, if the 25-rep technique still causes excessive pain, you may need to incorporate a partial range movement into the process. Start with the range that doesn't cause you any issues and over the next few weeks gradually increase the range of motion. The Smith Machine is perfect for this.

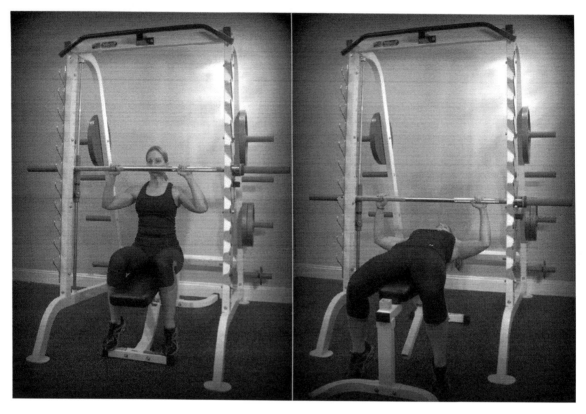

By using the safety catches, you can precisely manage the range of motion during rehab

Let's walk through this whole process using the RICE and Starr Recovery Protocol described above, in conjunction with the use of the Smith Machine. Let's assume one of your shoulders is bothering you when you bench press (an all too typical scenario). You had been bench pressing 225lbs for 6-8 reps for multiple sets when something went wrong.

For the first couple days, go see your doctor, take some anti-inflammatories and use the RICE technique. Assuming the doctor reports that nothing is seriously wrong and you really feel that to be the case, start using the Starr Recovery Protocol immediately. In our scenario, you should be performing three sets of bench presses using about 115lbs for 25 reps each set. Try using a full range of motion for the initial set of 25 reps. If the dull pain seems to subside as the set progresses, you should be fine with full range reps. Otherwise, set the safeties of the Smith Machine to a position where the pain diminishes as you perform those reps. Do this every day for the first two weeks, then re-evaluate your progress and decide if it's time to increase the range and weight and lower the reps. If things are progressing, that third week move to 125lbs for three sets of 20 reps on an every other day approach. For the fourth week, if things arc still progressing, go to 135lbs for three sets of 15 reps, following this protocol three times per week. From there, as long as everything is progressing nicely, continue the process. If at any point the injury seems to be staying the same or getting worse, go back a step or two and continue from there.

We're all different, every injury is unique and only you can honestly determine how you should apply the techniques above. In general, honesty, intelligence and patience will reward you here. Hubris, fear, and impatience will destroy you.

Handling Specific Injuries

Besides following the sound advice of RICE and Starr for rehab, there are some general tactics you can use to handle specific injuries. These include providing as much stability and pain-free range of motion on targeted exercises, especially in the early stages of recovery. That's why the Smith Machine can be a useful tool here—both of those things are built in. Another important consideration is to select appropriate exercises during rehab so you can continue training. Here's some specifics regarding common injuries.

Low Back Injuries

This is probably the most common type of injury, caused by anything from weak spinal erectors, tight hamstrings, failure to use periodization, rapidly picking up an all-too-heavy box left by UPS, shoveling snow (or dirt)—even sneezing. It happens—to all of us. Not only is this injury the most common, but it can also be the most humbling, especially if you find it difficult to use the bathroom and clean up your business.

To help recover from this type of injury try the following:

- Substitute Half Squats, Bench Squats, Bench Front Squats or Jefferson Squats for any full range squat movement in your workout.

- Substitute Sumo Deadlifts or Partial Deadlifts for regular Deadlifts.

- Substitute One-Arm Rows or Incline Bench Rows for Bent-Over Rows. This allows you to stabilize your body with your non-working arm or via the use of a bench.

- If the injury is recent or especially troubling, continue training your back with chinning movements. Chins should have almost no effect on your lower back.

To help prevent this type of injury in the future:

- Strengthen your abdominals with weighted Crunches.

- Incorporate Hanging Reverse Crunches into your program and become proficient at them.

- Consistently perform low back work, such as Deadlifts, Good Mornings, and Straight-Leg Deadlifts. This will strengthen your body's natural hinge movement.

- Lastly, but certainly not least, consistently stretch your hamstrings and lower back every day.

Shoulder Injuries

Let's talk about your shoulders next, because if your shoulders go, there goes pretty much the entire upper body. Because your shoulder complex is the only part of your body which is not directly supported by bones, it can be especially susceptible to strains and tears, and you'll need to be careful with all the soft tissues (muscles, tendons, and ligaments) holding things together. Usually, a shoulder injury only affects one side of the body and is often caused by sudden torque, excessive overload, chronic overuse, or imbalances between anterior (front) and posterior (rear) shoulder muscles—because everyone seems to be a pusher these days, it's likely the anterior pulling muscles of your shoulder are relatively weak.

To help recover from this type of injury try the following:

- Narrow your grip width when performing shoulder presses. Wider grip widths place additional stress on the connective structures of the shoulder, whereas narrower grips increase triceps involvement and reduce connective stressors. Find the right balance and grip width for your situation.

- Substitute Seated Military Presses for the standing variety—this increases stabilization and reduces the tendency to overwork the area with any push pressing initiatives.

- Substitute Seated Military Presses for the Press Behind the Neck. I've already discussed how that exercise is like navigating between Scylla and Charybdis, placing your shoulder structure into a razor's edge of effectiveness and doom, so you don't need to add that to your list of worries at this time.

- Substitute Seated Military Presses for Push Presses. Are you seeing the pattern here?

- In some cases, you may be able to press without shoulder pain by substituting Reverse Presses for your usual type of shoulder press. Try it.

- Use One-Arm Presses. This not only helps to work the injured shoulder but allows you to quickly assess any degree of asymmetry between both sides of your body.

- As Starr noted, Wide-Grip Upright Rows or High Pulls can exacerbate shoulder pain. If so, avoid these exercises until your shoulders allow you to resume.

- Use the Bent-Over Rear Delt Row. If this movement doesn't bother your shoulders, you need to keep at this useful movement to bring things back into balance.

To help prevent this type of injury in the future:

- Start with posterior shoulder movements first in your workout. This means any type of rowing exercise, including the Bent-Over Rear Delt Row.

- Group your shoulder work AFTER your chest or back work. Chest and back exercises indirectly warms, stretches and prepares the shoulders for direct action.

- Starr was right on the money on this one—high reps and low volume really help with shoulder recovery.

Knee Injuries

I see a lot of knee injuries from improper squatting technique (why is this so common?), particularly when the knee does not track in line with the foot position and direction. This type of injury can also occur with improper or inadequate warm-up. It's one thing to storm into the gym, lay down on the bench, and begin pressing (your shoulders will love you for that), and quite another to do the same with a squat movement. In the first case, you may be able to get away with that behavior in the short term if you're young, flexible and stupid, but the squat is a full-body movement and requires full-body prep.

To help recover from this type of injury try the following:

- Reduce the range of motion by performing Half Squats, Bench Squats, Bench Front Squats, or Jefferson Squats. But, really the best method for healing a knee injury is to follow Starr's high-rep protocol with full-range squats and light weight. Contrary to uninformed medical opinions or online personal trainer certificate holders, humans were designed to squat deeply and often. Over half the world does it on a daily basis for sustenance and survival.

- If only one knee is presenting an issue, omit any unilateral work (Step Ups, Lunges, Reverse Lunges, One-Leg Squats, and One-Leg Split Squats) from your routine and replace them with bilateral work—again, constantly monitoring the situation and ensuring that your form is not compensating in bad ways. Eventually, add the unilateral work back in with Starr as your guide.

To help prevent this type of injury in the future:

- Have someone who is proficient with squatting technique analyze your form for issues on a periodic basis (even the most experienced of us often get slightly untracked). If you don't have access to anyone like this, Bill Starr and Mark Rippetoe offer excellent articles, books and videos for reviewing proper form. It's often the person who is able to decompose issues and go back to the foundational core of the movement—no matter how many years you've been doing this weightlifting thing—that will overcome these types of obstacles and advance well past them.

- Warm up properly. If you ever get the chance to watch an accomplished competitive powerlifter press, squat or deadlift, you'll quickly notice a similar pattern. Even though these behemoths can lift 500+ pounds, typically they start warming up with just the bar. After that, only a couple plates are added for each subsequent warm-up set. Just because Ed Coan, arguably the world's greatest powerlifter, can squat over 800 pounds doesn't mean he starts warming up with 400.

- Stretch. In the 1980s, I remember watching professional bodybuilder Tom Platz, with legs larger than most men's waists, lie down on the floor, sink into a full split, *and then bend all the way backward*. Then, after a few minutes, he stood up, locked his legs straight and bent completely over until his head was between his legs (it was a tight fit). He talked of how the flexibility he developed over time greatly aided in his leg development. So, even if you don't want legs the size of five gallon buckets, incorporate stretching as a part of your daily routine. If you don't know how to stretch every part of your body, get yourself a copy of *Stretching*, by Bob Anderson. That book has been around for more than thirty years for good reason. It will teach you how to stretch properly. This is another one of those little things, like flossing your teeth, which you can do to live a healthier life.

- Ensure your knees track over your feet. If you notice your knees moving inward as you rise out of the bottom position of the squat, you likely have weak adductors, weak/tight hamstrings, or forgot the mental cue of *knees out*. To strengthen the adductor muscles, perform squatting movements with a wider than normal stance until the problem is corrected. Additionally, put as much effort into your hamstring training as you do for your quadriceps. If you are a parent and have more than one child—and you know this—it's not a good idea to play favorites. Most of these life lessons apply equally well in and out of the gym. Quadriceps and hamstrings are synergistic muscles—they need each other, and when called to action your hamstrings must be able to step up to the job.

Biceps, Elbow, and Forearm Injuries

Continuing our little journey through the land of common weight training injuries, we come to the dreaded biceps strain. This injury manifests itself as a dull pain around the lower part of your biceps or inner part of your forearm around the elbow. Besides overuse, this injury is typically caused by a sudden hyperextension when performing a curl. As Bill Pearl often said, we call this weight lifting, not weight throwing. There are two phases to weight lifting—the lifting part and the lowering part. Both are equally important. I see countless individuals concentrating on the former and not so much the latter. In the curl, after you've reached the top of the movement, surely you don't let the bar drop like someone cut the cord on an elevator. If it takes you two seconds to lift the weight, make sure it takes at least the same amount of time to lower it. Remember our symphony analogy and tempo. In his book, *Loaded Guns*, former Mr. Olympia Larry Scott relates how the starting and ending position of the curl is where all the gold is in that exercise. He was talking about the importance of starting and ending that movement with great exertion, under complete control and with immaculate form. Nowhere is form more critical than at the start of the exercise and as you approach the end of the movement. Where there be gold, there also be dragons. This lesson applies to any movement.

To help recover from this type of injury try the following:

- Because this type of injury is often the result of overuse, sometimes the best thing to do is to rest the area or at least refrain from direct biceps and forearm work. Don't worry—if you're performing deadlifts, rows, and chins, those biceps aren't going anywhere.

- Make sure you use an overhand grip on deadlifts, rows and chins. Now is not the time to directly stress the biceps with an underhand or reverse grip.

- If you have Close-Grip Pull-Ups in your routine, substitute Curls or Drag Curls because they place proportionately less stress on the biceps tendon and the elbows.

- For some, extensions will aggravate the elbow area. If you find yourself in this camp, omit extensions until the injury has healed. You should probably be doing more Close-Grip Bench Presses anyway.

To help prevent this type of injury in the future:

- Yes, you can beat a dead horse, so I'm going to do it again. Warm up those elbows before working out. Light, high-rep pushdowns work well here.

- Change your grip width periodically. Just like so many other things, if you keep doing something time and again, your body will either adapt to it, or start to break. Tendonitis of the elbow is a warning sign that your elbow structure is starting to tear. Periodic rest and change are your dual knights to keep that foe at bay.

Calf Injuries

Some of us relish the almost pleasurable pain of sore calves. Unlike other muscle soreness, you can't escape this one, because it sticks its calling card in your face with every step you take. Call us masochists.

However, that's not what we're talking about here.

I'm referring to a strain of your Achilles tendon area, typically caused by a hyperextension on calf raises (stretching your calves too far, too suddenly).

To help recover from this type of injury try the following:

- Limit the range of motion on Calf Raises (seated, standing, kneeling, or Donkey varieties) by standing directly on the floor—don't elevate your toes on plates, aerobic steps, etc. We want to ensure that you start from the same foot position as walking.

To help prevent this type of injury in the future:

- Always warm-up your calf muscles by performing some simple body weight raises both in the standing and seated positions.

- Control the negative, lowering portion of all calf raise movements. The most common way people injure their calves is by rushing through the movement, in some perverse sort of rapid-fire machination, that often evokes both poor form and subsequently produces little results. Remember, we lift weights, we do not ballistically throw them.

Neck Injuries

Whether you've ever worked out with weights before or not, everyone's had a sore neck at some point. Usually you discover this after waking up from sleeping for several hours with your head hanging off the pillow (or bed) and you can't turn your head much (if at all) without pain. Well, in the gym it can happen much faster and often you know you've strained your neck or trapezius muscles with that sudden movement under load.

To help recover from this type of injury try the following:

- Eliminate any exercises that involve the neck musculature or surrounding area until healed. This includes Shrugs, Upright Rows, High Pulls, Deadlifts, and possibly any shoulder presses. If it's just a simple sprain, your neck will heal quickly in a matter of days. But, of course, your doctor will know this more accurately than you or I.

To help prevent this type of injury in the future:

- Don't move your head during an exercise. You aren't going for a power walk or jogging through the neighborhood or turning your head to talk to your lifting buddy or the pretty girl/guy next to you. You are lifting weights, maybe substantial weights, which place a load on not only the target muscle(s), but the entire musculoskeletal system. Things under load are wary of sudden movement.

8

Intensity Techniques

Some have said that intensity is a young man's game. To that I counter with, do you feel young at heart? That may be more important as you read through this section and determine your path.

As the great philosopher (and former heavyweight boxing champion) Mike Tyson has said, "Everybody's got a plan—until they get hit." Even if you follow the best weight training plan for your desired goal with consistency and conviction, eventually, even the best of us will reach a limit to how much weight we are able to lift in a particular exercise. The glory days of linear progression have come to a halt. Our workouts don't seem to work anymore. Now, you need to change something to make the body adapt. Often, desperate times do call for desperate measures. That's where intensity techniques come into play. Think of them as your desperate measures, those nuclear weight training options. Just like Mike, you'll need to learn to bob and weave with these techniques, interlacing them with your prescribed plans, in order to deliver that well-timed blow that will propel your body back into adaptation mode. Muscle growth must often be shoved forward, not coerced.

There are a myriad of intensity enhancing techniques you can apply to your workouts, but here I'm just going to present the ones that take advantage of the Smith Machine's strengths. Most of them adjust the variables of distance, time, and volume.

Here are the intensity techniques I'll discuss that are well-suited to the strengths of the Smith Machine:

- **Rest-Pause**
- **Drop-Sets**
- **Static Holds**
- **Partials**
- **Negatives**

Now, lets's look at each one in detail.

Rest-Pause

This technique allows you to extend a set by taking extremely short rest intervals (5-15 seconds) between reps as you approach failure. In practice, performing two rest-pauses during your set should work best. Rest-Pause works extremely well on the Smith Machine because you can easily rack the bar at any point and then continue, without fear of the weight falling on you.

Although you'll typically use this technique as you approach failure, you can also use it right from the start of a set, in order to handle some really heavy weights.

Here's an example of a Rest-Pause set of Smith Machine bench presses: **225x8+2+1**

In this example, we managed 8 reps with 225lbs, racked the bar in the machine for about 10 seconds, did another 2 reps, racked it again, and then did a final rep, for a total of 11 reps in the rest-pause set. Much more intense than if we just did 225 for 8 reps and called it a set.

Partials

The great strongman Paul Anderson helped propel the use of partial reps to the forefront of strength training in the 1950s. Although Mr. Anderson may have initiated this technique by standing in a hole in the ground with a tractor axle on his back for squats—slowly filling in the hole as he became stronger (and thus increasing the range of motion)—you can accomplish much the same with the Smith Machine.

Partial reps (Partials) use only a limited range of the full range of motion for an exercise. This allows you to use more weight than usual, thus increasing the stress (load) on the muscle as well as providing the stimulus to build stronger connective tissue (tendons and ligaments). Along with Negatives, they are especially effective for breaking through weight plateaus.

Other than a traditional power rack, the Smith Machine coupled with its safety catches is just about the perfect way to perform partials safely. If you are executing partials right from the get go, set the safety catches to hold the bar at the lowest position of the range you want to work. If you are doing partials at the end of a normal range set, adjust the safety catches to the lowest position of the full range—this way you won't get stuck if you go to complete muscular failure.

Partials can be performed anywhere within an exercise's range of motion—get creative with this. You can also perform them at the end of a set, when you can't complete another full range of motion with the exercise.

So, what's a recommended number of partials to perform at the end of a set? Try for 3-6 and see how that works for you.

Some good examples of using partials on the Smith Machine include:

Back

I don't recommend the use of partial movements for the back, other than partial deadlifts (Rack Pulls). The back really needs full range of motion to grow to its full potential.

Chest

Adjust the safety catches so that you can perform only the top portion of the press—or the mid-range of the press—or the start of the press. You get the idea. By the way, this is a proven technique to increase your bench press.

Thighs (Quadriceps)

Adjust the safety catches so that you perform only the top part of the squat, as in Half Squats.

Calves

At the end of your set of calf raises perform just the bottom half of the motion. For seated raises, try performing just the top half of the motion.

Drop Sets

Drop sets require you to perform a set of an exercise to failure (or just short of failure), then reduce the weight slightly and continue the set for additional reps. This technique is designed to build muscle mass and endurance, and is not as effective for building strength, power, or speed. Because you can quickly remove plates from the Smith Machine, drop sets work particularly well here.

The theory behind drop sets is that even though you may have reached a point of positive muscular failure, you may not have activated all your muscle fiber types in that area. You can recruit additional fibers by continuing the set through immediate weight reductions, thus increasing the stress and overload placed on the muscle, forcing adaptation to occur.

So, one question you may have is—how much should I reduce (drop) the weight each time? Good question. A common method is to reduce the weight about 15% for each "drop", although the real answer is you'll need to experiment to find out the best amount based on your current capabilities. Eventually, you may discover that your drop weight percentage goes down (a good thing), because your muscular endurance is improving.

In order to maximize the efficiency of drop sets, keep these key points in mind:

- **Set up your equipment in advance** (with the Smith Machine, we're all set up!)

- **Keep rest intervals to a minimum** (1-10 seconds between weight drops, so you need to move fast when changing weights.) Remember, the shorter the rest interval, the higher the intensity.

- **Perform two weight drops** (most of the time)

- **Perform 4-6 reps per drop** (again, most of the time)

- **Use drop sets sparingly**

There are many variations of drop sets, so let's look at those.

Ascending Drop Sets

Decrease the weight by a substantial amount and increase the number of reps at each drop. A typical rep pattern here is 6-12-20 (6 reps with initial weight, 12 reps after first drop, and 20 reps with the final drop). This technique starts powerfully and builds to a lactic acid crescendo.

Descending Drop Sets (Tight Drop Sets)

Decrease the weight by a small amount so that the number of reps at each drop decreases. A typical rep pattern here is 12-8-4-2. This is an example of a Tight Drop Set.

Grip/Stance Change Drop Sets

Change your grip or foot stance width between each weight drop. The purpose here is to subject the muscle(s) to stress from differing angles and load patterns.

This technique is particularly effective with barbell rows, bench presses and squats.

Halves

Reduce the weight by 50% between drops. This will allow you to start with a heavy weight that you can manage for a few reps and lets you keep going into the higher reps as the weight lightens.

Halves work really well for the big lifts, like squats, presses and rows. Also, try them with drag curls and calf raises (your calves will love you for this one).

Power Drop Sets

This variation combines heavy weights, low reps, and small drops in weight (10-15%). Try to keep the reps at six on each drop and just perform two drops.

If you did this for bench presses, it would look like this:

Smith Machine Bench Press: 275x6 > 245x6 > 205x6

Rest-Pause Drop Sets

This is a classic technique used by many competitive bodybuilders. After reaching a point just short of failure, rest for a fixed number of seconds (five, ten, or fifteen) between drops. This allows your muscles to slightly recover—therefore, you can use more weight with this technique, which is why it's good for increasing strength and size.

Strip Sets

This is where the plates are "stripped" off the barbell as the set progresses. This is what most people think of when we talk about drop sets.

Try this one with presses, starting with a bunch of 10lb plates on each side of the bar. By the time all the plates are removed, that empty bar is going to feel awfully heavy.

Wide Drop Sets

This variation refers to large weight reductions between drops. Wide drop sets are typically easier to perform than tight drop sets, because they allow you to perform higher reps. Due to the higher reps and subsequent cardiovascular fatigue, wide drop sets are particularly useful for exercises that work large muscle groups, such as chest, back and legs.

Try these with presses and squats.

Here's an example of a wide drop set: **Smith Machine Bench Press: 275x5 > 205x12 > 135x20**

Negatives

This technique concentrates on the eccentric (lowering) phase of the exercise. It's typical to perform Negatives at the end of a set, when your muscles have failed from performing the exercise. However, you can perform Negatives effectively as standalone sets.

There are a couple points to keep in mind in order to perform Negatives effectively on the Smith Machine:

- Don't perform negatives unless you are an advanced weight trainer. These are brutal to execute and beginners don't have the systemic adaptation to handle this yet.

- Use a weight that's about 10% heavier than your one-rep max (1RM) on the exercise

- Actively resist the lowering of the weight the entire time. Make gravity earn every inch of movement.

- The negative rep should take about 5-10 seconds to lower—if it descends faster than that on the first negative then the weight is too heavy.

- Try to perform negatives near the beginning of your workouts (after warm-ups and some working sets, of course) when you are at full energy. Negatives can sap energy like nothing else.

- Don't perform negatives at every workout, because they can create extreme stress on the body. This technique will test your body's recovery ability to the limit.

Static Holds

This technique is as much for your mind as your body and is one of the places in weight training where you learn to confront your fear. It's simple. After a couple of regular sets of an exercise, pick a weight heavier than anything you've ever performed with that exercise. Then, just hold it in the contracted position as long as possible.

Static Holds will help to build connective tissue strength, increase muscle density and improve your confidence with heavy weights. You can also use this technique at various stages of an exercise's range of motion in order to break through performance plateaus.

Best used with compound, multi-joint movements such as presses, squats, and deadlifts, the Smith Machine is definitely your friend here. Use the safety catches to set the position you want to perform the Static Hold in, and then go for it.

So, how much weight should you use? Try anywhere from 10-50% more weight than you can handle with a normal range of motion.

Here's a tip: use Static Holds (no wrist straps allowed!) to build both big forearms and bigger traps/neck. Just set the safety catches a couple inches below your bottom range for shrugs so that when your grip gives out, everybody stays safe.

9

Beyond the Smith Machine

Once you understand how to effectively use the Smith Machine, the key point to remember during your life-long fitness odyssey is that nothing works forever and everything works for a short time.

So, on those days when you're not rushed for time, when the gym is less crowded and plateaus are on the horizon, injuries remain at bay, and when you have the confidence and courage to venture forth, I hope you walk right past that Smith Machine and grab the sure steel of barbells and dumbbells. Suddenly, the universe will seem vast, but your navigation true. That is your way forward.

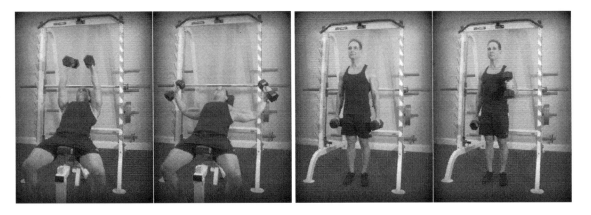

You can't perform natural arc-based or neutral-grip movementss on the Smith Machine

The final lesson here, and it's a good one both inside and outside the gym, is not to stay anchored in the safe harbor of the past, physically or mentally—that's the recipe for mediocrity, stagnation and eventual failure.

Remember—if the conditions warrant, the Smith Machine will always remain as a companion on your journey. Godspeed.

Where to go from here

I hope this book has introduced or expanded your knowledge, thirst and desire regarding weight training. For a book about the Smith Machine, it may seem counterintuitive to encourage you to apply this knowledge to free weights, but that is what I hope you do. Although the past half century has witnessed numerous exercise inventions and apparatus of dubious and useful nature, nothing, and I mean nothing, has ever been able to succeed and produce the speed, magnitude and ferocity of results that the mighty barbell and its kindred dumbbell or kettlebell can illicit.

In that vein, here are some guideposts for your further travel down those roads.

Strength Training

In the world of barbell-based strength training, you can't go wrong by reading any material by Bill Starr, Mark Rippetoe and Dan John. These will get you started.

- *Only the Strongest Shall Survive: Strength Training for Football*, Bill Starr.
- *Starting Strength*, Mark Rippetoe.
- *Practical Programming for Strength Training*, Mark Rippetoe.
- *Never Let Go: A Philosophy of Lifting, Living and Learning*, Dan John.

Bodybuilding & Hypertrophy-Based Training

What you don't want to do here is pick up one of the numerous bodybuilding magazines at the supermarket or convenience store. Besides simply being a pictorially glorified catalog of mostly useless nutritional supplements, accompanied by pictures of chemically enhanced physiques, they contain little actual information that stray from the volume training approach. For the cost of about three of these magazines, you could purchase one of the books below that will provide you with a vast expanse of knowledge that will last a lifetime.

The names you are looking for here are John McCallum, Bill Pearl, Dave Draper, Stuart McRobert and Clarence Bass.

- *The Complete Keys to Progress*, John McCallum.
- *Keys to the Inner Universe*, Bill Pearl.
- *Brother Iron, Sister Steel: A Bodybuilder's Book*, Dave Draper.
- Any of the *Brawn* series of books by Stuart McRobert.
- Any of the *Ripped* series of books by Clarence Bass.

Additionally, I'll refer you to one of my other books, *Bodybuilding: From Heavy Duty to SuperSlow*, because I think it's the best overview of all the various bodybuilding training systems of the past century ever written. In fact, at the time of this writing, it's the only one. That's why I wrote it. Get a quick lesson on all your bodybuilding training options, and then pick the one that fits your interest, time, age, genetics and situation.

Circuit Training, Weak Point Training, and Injury Rehab

Pearl, Draper and Bass provide ample information and ideas regarding training with minimal rest and circuit training in their books. All of the books above address weak points through balanced approaches to increasing strength and size. And, as I've mentioned previously, the Starr book provides the most in-depth discussion of injury rehab and recovery, including actual case studies, that I've ever read.

Read all of the books listed above and you'll know more than almost anyone else you'll ever meet in a gym. Now, you just have to go apply it.

Afterword

I lied. Please forgive me.

In the beginning of this book I told you it was written for two audiences—those relative beginners using primarily exercise machines, and the more experienced weight trainers looking for another tool to help them further along on their journey.

This book is really a Trojan horse.

Years ago, I finally convinced my father to join a gym and start working out. He's actually stuck with it, although he's never ventured beyond the rudimentary selectorized machines. My father has had genetically high hypertension for most of his life, something he passed to me. Luckily, modern medicine keeps such things at bay. But no one likes to see their parents age, and ultimately decline physically and die. We search for anything that can keep their quality of life high and them with us a little longer. Although not the eternal fountain of youth, weight training can often slow the hands of time for many. As Jack Lalanne originally envisioned, if the Smith Machine can be used as an inviting tool to further guide someone towards sound weight training techniques, principles and possibilities, along with improved health, I'm going to use it. As I wrote this book, I often asked myself how would I explain a particular exercise or concept to my father. This book is for you, dad.

We all have fathers, mothers, brothers and sisters, sons and daughters, and friends we love. Weight training may be one avenue to keep them around longer and provide them with a higher quality of life. Hopefully, they even come to love it, as I have. If you know someone who shows any interest in improving their health and fitness, and you think this book may help them towards that goal, please give them a copy. The lessons here transcend the machine.

God bless.

Craig
July 2013

About the Author

Craig Cecil has been involved in sports and the science of exercise since his days of high school athletics in baseball, through his collegiate career in NCAA Track & Field, to his devotion to weightlifting and bodybuilding pursuits over the past 20 years. During that time, Craig has trained with professional athletes, as well as multitudes of dedicated, ordinary individuals just wanting to build lean, muscular body weight. Craig is a member of the National Strength & Conditioning Association and holds an MBA from Loyola University of Maryland.

Other Books by Craig Cecil

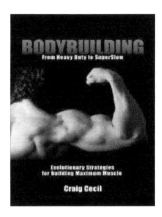

Bodybuilding: From Heavy Duty to SuperSlow

Bodybuilding: From Heavy Duty to SuperSlow takes you through the evolution of bodybuilding training, from early 20th century circus strongmen to the latest muscle-building techniques of today. Learn how to harness these concepts to build muscle faster than you thought possible.

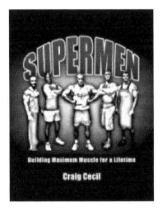

Supermen: Building Maximum Muscle for a Lifetime

Supermen: Building Maximum Muscle for a Lifetime presents a weightlifting system for intermediate to advanced weight trainers that maximize the muscular development of an individual, while creating a complete, balanced and symmetrical physique. This book will save you years of trial-and-error in the gym and provide you with decades of weight training insights. It's a book for the rest of us—those with average genetics, strong minds and stronger hearts.

42538696R00208

Made in the USA
San Bernardino, CA
05 December 2016